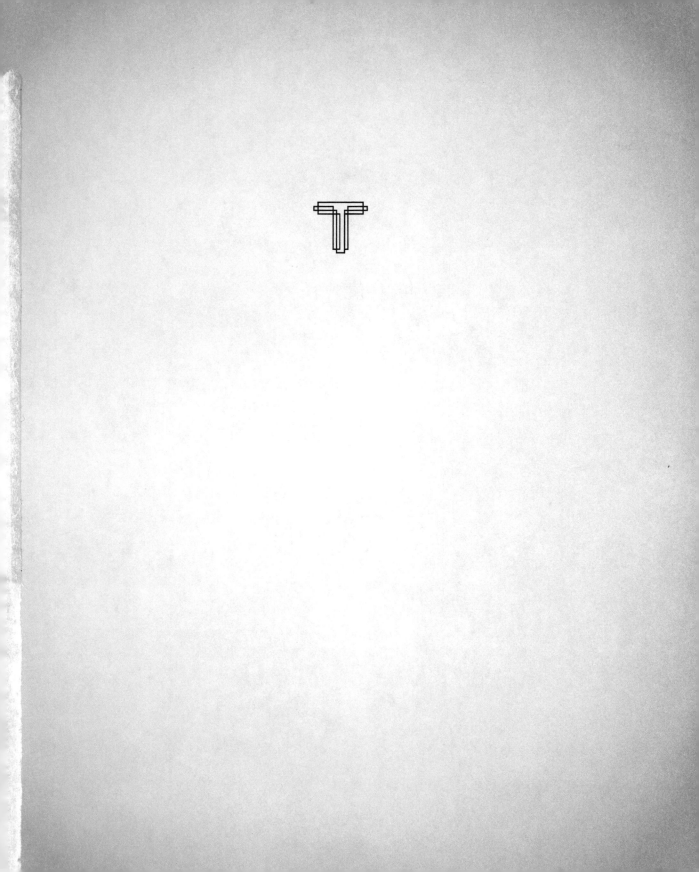

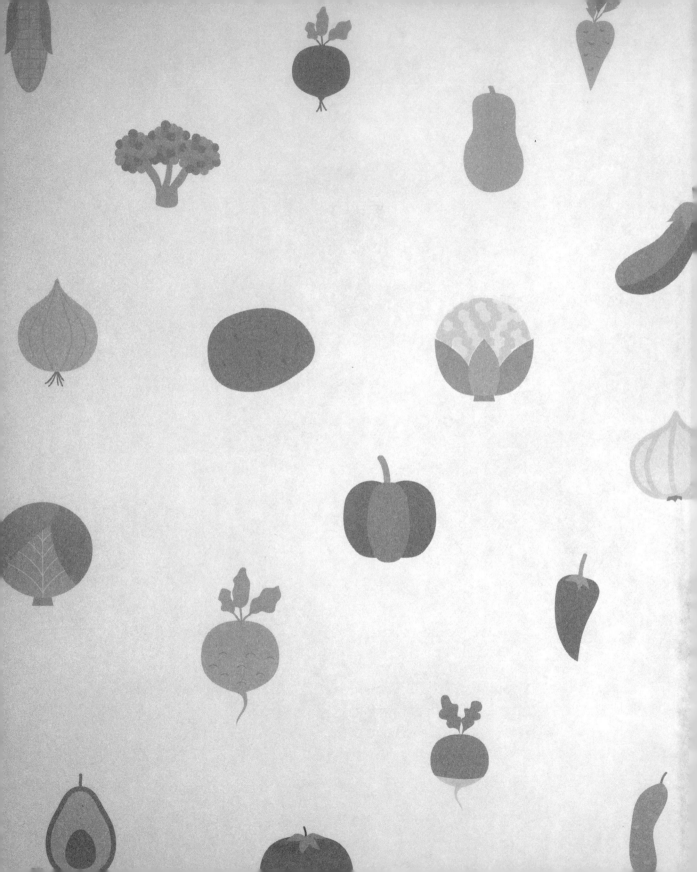

FORKS
OVER KNIVES®
FAMILY

Every Parent's Guide
to Raising Healthy,
Happy Kids on a
Whole-Food, Plant-Based Diet

Alona Pulde, MD, and Matthew Lederman, MD, with Marah Stets and Brian Wendel
Recipes by Darshana Thacker

Touchstone

New York   London   Toronto   Sydney   New Delhi

Touchstone
An Imprint of Simon & Schuster, Inc.
1230 Avenue of the Americas
New York, NY 10020

Copyright © 2016 by Forks Over Knives, LLC
Photographs copyright © 2016 by Matt Armendariz

First Touchstone hardcover edition September 2016

TOUCHSTONE and colophon are registered trademarks of Simon & Schuster, Inc.

For information about special discounts for bulk purchases,
please contact Simon & Schuster Special Sales at 1-866-506-1949
or business@simonandschuster.com.

The Simon & Schuster Speakers Bureau can bring authors to your live event.
For more information or to book an event, contact the Simon & Schuster Speakers Bureau
at 1-866-248-3049 or visit our website at www.simonspeakers.com.

Manufactured in the United States of America

1   3   5   7   9   10   8   6   4   2

Library of Congress Cataloging-in-Publication Data

Names: Pulde, Alona, author. | Lederman, Matthew, author. |
Stets, Marah, author. | Wendel, Brian, author.
Title: Forks over knives family : every parent's guide to raising
healthy, happy kids on a whole-food, plant-based diet / Alona Pulde, MD,
Matthew Lederman, MD, With Marah Stets, And Brian Wendel ; Recipes by Darshana Thacker.
Description: New York : Touchstone Books, 2016. | Includes bibliographical references and index.
Identifiers: LCCN 2016011411 | ISBN 9781476753324 (hardcover) | ISBN 9781476753331 (pbk.)
Subjects: LCSH: Natural foods—Health aspects. | Veganism—Health aspects. | Cooking
(Natural foods) | Children—Nutrition. | LCGFT: Cookbooks.
Classification: LCC RM237.55 .P84 2016 | DDC 641.5/637—dc23
LC record available at https://lccn.loc.gov/2016011411

ISBN 978-1-4767-5332-4
ISBN 978-1-4767-5334-8 (ebook)

We dedicate this book to all the courageous families who dare to step away from what is comfortable and customary to seek better and healthier ways of living, for themselves and for their children.

And to Kylee and Jordan, who motivate us every day to stay on our path. Watching them grow healthy and well is the most rewarding gift of all.

CONTENTS

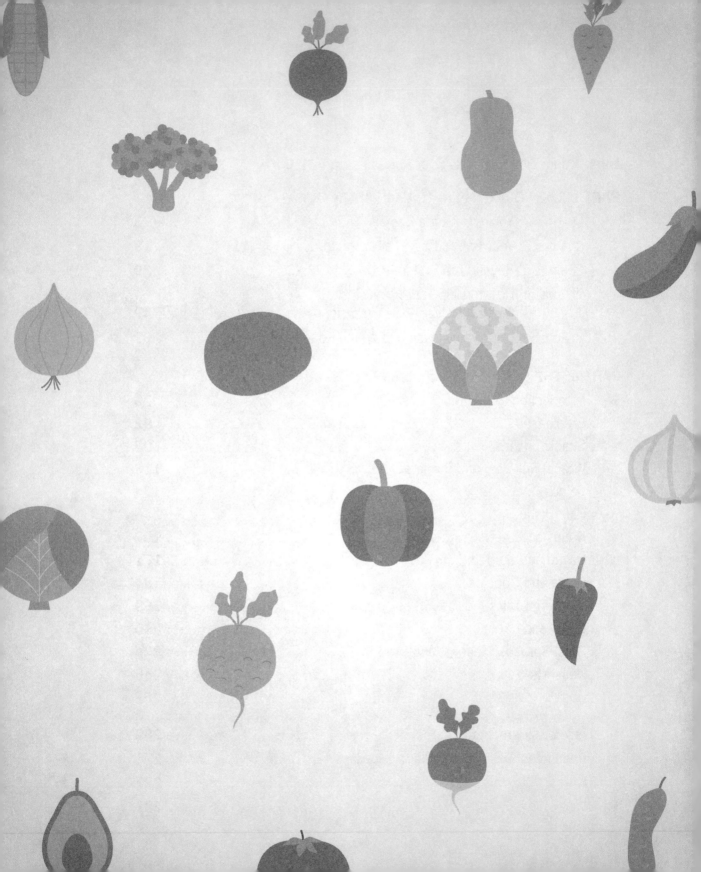

Introduction:
Why the *Forks Over Knives Family?*

Every year, more and more people learn about the enormous benefits of a whole-food, plant-based lifestyle. Millions of men and women have learned that simply by eating well they can prevent and even reverse disease, increase their vitality and strength, improve mental clarity, and reach an ideal weight. Perhaps you recently made this discovery yourself and have just begun to eat this way. Or maybe you've been living the Forks Over Knives way for many years. You might be thinking about starting a family and want to know what to expect during your plant-based pregnancy and your baby's first year. Or you may already have older children and need the tools to help everyone in your house transition to the whole-food, plant-based lifestyle. Wherever you are on your own journey, you are there because you understand that the food-as-medicine concept isn't only about *your* gaining the best possible health for yourself. It's about making changes that will help the whole family achieve and maintain the best possible health—not just for now, but for a lifetime.

In our previous book, *The Forks Over Knives Plan*, we explained in great detail why a whole-food, plant-based diet is the optimum choice a person can make for him- or herself. We also laid out a program to fully transition to the lifestyle in about a month. If you'd like more information on the research behind this way of eating and a week-by-week plan for transitioning, we encourage you to refer to that book.

This book is a little different, and we were moved to write it first and foremost by our experiences as doctors. For years we ran a medical practice using this diet as a primary treatment, and we continue to counsel people daily on how to implement or maintain the lifestyle. We have been privileged to see countless success stories manifest right before our eyes, not only for our patients but very often for their families, too. We love the opportunity to work one-on-one with so many people, but the world is vast and we're impatient to reach as many others as we can. This book is our chance to help *you* apply these changes in your own life. Whether you're brand-new to this way of eating or you're already eating a whole-food, plant-based diet yourself, the fact is that it becomes easier for everybody when the whole family is doing it.

There are two other, very important reasons for our writing this book, and they are at the heart of our nonprofessional lives: Kylee and Jordan, our beautiful little girls. When we started our whole-food, plant-based journey we did not have children, and now that we do, we are even more profoundly grateful that we discovered the lifestyle and are raising our girls this way. We've certainly faced many of the challenges that come with having plant-based children in a Standard American Diet world. Just like parents everywhere, we're learning along the way, and we hope that some of what we've learned can be useful to you and make your path a little smoother.

We are grateful and delighted for the opportunity to share what we know as doctors *and* as parents in this book, with which we aim to make living a whole-food, plant-based lifestyle with a family not only manageable but also as joyful and as tasty as it can be. We jump in to the hands-on advice in Chapter 1, but first we will briefly outline the basic concepts of the diet. Whether you are very familiar with the lifestyle or it's entirely new to you, reviewing the Forks Over Knives foundation in this section will allow you to read without scratching your head when we refer to these key principles throughout the book:

- The definition of the whole-food, plant-based diet

- Focus on the best food "package"

- Calorie density

- The Dopamine Pleasure Cycle

- Identifying and meeting your personal needs

THE WHOLE-FOOD, PLANT-BASED DIET DEFINED

There is a lot of misconception about what a whole-food, plant-based diet is, so we want to begin by clearly defining this term. We find that even people with some familiarity with the diet still sometimes believe that we eat (and are raising our children on!) primarily leafy greens and carrots. In fact, in this lifestyle you'll be eating foods like burritos, lasagna, mashed potatoes, hearty casseroles, and stews. These delectable meals may be prepared a little differently—without dairy and oil, for example—but nonetheless you will find that you are eating the same hearty comfort food you've long been used to. To make these delicious meals, you will be choosing foods from these categories:

- Fruits (apples, blueberries, mangoes, etc.)

- Vegetables (carrots, broccoli, collards, etc.)

- Tubers and starchy vegetables (potatoes, corn, winter squash, etc.)

- Whole grains (brown rice, oats, quinoa, etc.)

- Legumes (black beans, chickpeas, lentils, etc.)

There is one important point to stress, and it's vital to making the lifestyle work over the long term. The center of your plate must be a starch food, such as those under tubers and starchy vegetables, whole grains, or legumes in the list above. (You can also make a meal out of fruit, but you will need to eat an especially generous portion.) The reason is simple: leafy vegetables alone do not contain enough calories to make a meal. Your family and growing children will not find a meal of leafy salads or steamed veggies very satisfying. That is to say, they may temporarily find it pleasing, but in a short time they will be hungry again, and people can't live in this sort of cycle for very long. In fact, we find that one reason some people don't stick with the whole-food, plant-based lifestyle is that they actually try to live primarily on vegetables, or even on vegetables alone. This is a mistake. We *need* to eat whole, minimally processed carbohydrates; they are not only good for us, they also fill us up. So eat your starch!

If you've tried and failed to implement other "diets" and "healthy eating plans" in your house, you're likely to find the whole-food, plant-based way of eating more straightforward than what has come before. There is no need to follow specific, rigid guidelines on what to eat and when to eat it. All you need to do is prepare your meals and eat generously from the foods listed on the previous page. If you need inspiration, we can't think of a better place to begin than the recipes in this book, which start on page 92.

THERE'S NO SUCH THING AS EATING FOR SINGLE NUTRIENTS; IT'S THE PACKAGE THAT COUNTS

There is a popular misconception that we can eat in a way that targets individual nutrients—and even that we *should* eat this way. However, there is no benefit to eating any specific food in order to get one or another nutrient. No food contains only a single nutrient; food has countless nutrients. What matters most is a food's *overall* nutrient profile, or "package." Animal-based and processed foods provide packages with a disproportionate amount of nutrients, so that we get much more than we actually need (such as too much acidic protein), as well as an abundance of harmful substances (such as cholesterol in animal foods), which we don't need to consume at all. Other problems include being devoid of important nutrients such as fiber and certain vitamins and minerals.

What's worse, many of the foods often singled out as good sources for nutrients are some of the most damaging to human health because they come in these terrible packages. For instance, many people consume lots of dairy and meat in a quest for calcium and protein to build strong bones. However, evidence shows that this can actually increase the risk of osteoporosis and kidney stones.[1] In fact, one excellent review article concluded that "osteoporotic bone fracture rates are highest in countries that consume the most dairy, calcium, and animal protein" and that "most studies of fracture risk provide little or no evidence that milk or other dairy products benefit bone."[2] Whole, plant-based food, on the other hand, provides the best package of nutrients—and in proportions that are most consistent with human needs.

In spite of abundant evidence, this misconception about eating foods for nutrients is not limited to people eating the Standard American Diet. Even people on a plant-based regimen, especially parents with children, sometimes worry about getting enough of some nutrient or another, and they will try to target specific foods—such as certain green vegetables for calcium, beans for protein, and so on. If this sounds familiar, you can abandon that kind of thinking. The most important and the very best thing you can do for yourself and for your family is simply to use the foods from the categories on page xi to prepare dishes that you all will love. In most cases, it is more important to simply eat whole plant foods than spend time focusing on which whole plant foods you eat.

IT'S ABOUT CALORIE DENSITY, *NOT* CALORIE COUNTING

One of the great advantages of eating a whole-food, plant-based diet is that there is no need to count calories or practice portion control. On the Standard American Diet, the only way to maintain weight is through portion control. On a whole-food, plant-based diet, you can control weight *without* portion control—and you optimize your health.

To understand why this is true, it helps to first understand how hunger signals work in the body. We must eat a certain quantity of food at each meal before our stomach stretches enough to signal our brain that we have reached satiety and can stop eating. Whole, plant-based foods have more bulk than animal-based and processed foods because they contain more water and fiber. They literally fill our stomachs more, which shuts down those hunger signals. A whole-food, plant-based diet is the only way to eat enough to feel satiated while consuming fewer calories. The reason for this lies in the *calorie density* of the food you eat. Calorie density is the number of calories in a given weight of food, usually expressed as calories per pound. Leafy vegetables have 100 to 200 calories per pound, and tubers and starchy vegetables have 300 to 400 calories per pound. Meat, on the other hand, contains about 1,200 calories per pound, and oil contains roughly 4,000 calories per pound.

Foods with a high calorie density tend to take up less space in your stomach, so you will tend to consume more calories than you need to feel full. (Note, though, that foods too *low* in calorie density tend to take up more space in your stomach, so you typically consume fewer calories than you need in order to feel full. This is what happens when you try to eat just fruits and vegetables; you simply won't have the time or desire to eat enough food to meet your caloric needs.) The ideal is the middle "sweet spot," a diet with a healthy average of about 550 calories per pound. And, in fact, a diet based on fruits and vegetables, as well as tubers and starchy vegetables, whole grains, and legumes—in other words, the Forks Over Knives whole-food, plant-based diet—will average around 550 calories per pound and will provide your body the appropriate volume of food to signal you have had enough to eat. This means that when you eat whole, plant-based foods, your body will reach satiation with many fewer calories—without your ever needing to count a single one.

Calorie Density for Common Foods

Here are the calorie densities (approximate calories in 1 pound) for a variety of common foods:

Raw and leafy vegetables	70–200
Fruits	200–400
Tubers and starchy vegetables	300–400
Whole grains	400–500
Legumes	500–600
Whole-wheat pasta, cooked	550
Avocado	750
Whole-wheat bread	1,150
Meat	1,200
Pure sugar	1,800
Chocolate	2,200
Nuts and seeds	2,600
Oils	4,000

THE DOPAMINE PLEASURE CYCLE

Being hungry for or even craving a specific food is a natural part of the human experience. We crave certain foods based on how stimulating they are (i.e., how much dopamine they trigger the release of). And this ultimately translates into making us feel better emotionally and physically. However, it is important to note that this is not because we have an actual biological need for the food in question; it's because of the Dopamine Pleasure Cycle. When we eat, the chemical dopamine is released in our brain, which gives us a pleasurable sensation that makes us want to eat more. This is a survival mechanism to make sure we eat. The more refined or calorie-dense a food is, the greater the dopamine hit.[3] This worked great for our ancestors, because when they required energy, the craving for calorie richness would make them choose, for example, bananas over nonstarchy vegetables. Bananas are sufficiently caloric to make a meal of, while nonstarchy vegetables on their own are not, so being wired this way made good sense for survival.

However, this natural preference for highly rich foods gets us in trouble today, since the choices are no longer limited to healthy foods such as bananas and leafy greens. The presence of highly processed food and the abundance of meats are game changers. These rich foods, by exceeding the calorie density of the fruit and starches we thrive on, "trick" our senses and give us a hyper-normal amount of pleasure. For example, if you were to put a chocolate fudge cake and an orange next to each other, most of us would gravitate to the chocolate cake. The higher calorie density of the cake makes it more pleasurable, despite the fact that it doesn't support health the way an orange does.

Furthermore, the more artificially rich foods we eat, the more our bodies crave them and the less satisfying healthy foods are by comparison. We even begin to depend on this artificially heightened level of pleasure and can experience a "high" feeling because the dopamine hit in our brain is the same as if we were taking drugs. Our friend Doug Lisle, PhD, calls this "the Pleasure Trap." * Too many people think that if they just tried harder and had more "willpower," they'd be able to have these foods in moderation. But the truth is that the solution is not "trying harder" or "controlling yourself"; it is, instead, the whole-food, plant-based diet. When you detach yourself from (and continue to avoid) the Dopamine Pleasure Cycle, your body remembers how to respond to the real food you were designed to eat.

IDENTIFY AND MEET YOUR OWN NEEDS

Meeting your own needs can be easy to forget in the hustle and bustle of family life, but we all have them—even busy parents! We are most successful at any endeavor when we can identify what our needs are and how best to meet

---

* Many of the precepts in this section come from *The Pleasure Trap: Mastering the Hidden Force That Undermines Health & Happiness* by Douglas J. Lisle, PhD, and Alan Goldhamer, DC.

them, ideally not at the expense of others. When it comes to diet and lifestyle change, we have found that four primary personal needs come up most often:

- Health: You need to feel vital, strong, happy, and well.

- Pleasure: You need to feel good and enjoy what you eat.

- Ease: You need living and eating healthy to be easy—and not take up too much of your precious resources of time or money.

- Acceptance: You need your family, friends, and colleagues and your larger circle of community to accept how you live and eat, even if you make different choices than they do.

Consider how you would order these needs from most to least important and think about how you can meet each one. No matter what your needs are or how you prioritize them, the beauty of the whole-food, plant-based lifestyle is that all can be met by the diet. You can have good health; eat delicious, easy-to-prepare food (the recipes in this book will get you started); and share all of it with your family and larger community.

The important thing is not to lose sight of your personal needs and to realize that how you rank them and endeavor to meet them now may be different from how it will be in a few months. This is perfectly normal. Just remember to check in with yourself (and your family; see page 48) from time to time. And when you encounter challenges and obstacles, as you surely will, focus less on the problems themselves and more on what lies behind them. The answer will almost always be found first by figuring out which of your needs aren't being met, and second by strategizing how to resolve them.

HOW TO USE THIS BOOK

In this book we focus on practical, hands-on advice for living the whole-food, plant-based way with your family. It doesn't matter where in life you are—whether as a parent or as a follower of the lifestyle. Our advice and guidance covers every stage of parenting—from pregnancy to raising teenagers—and it doesn't matter if you're new to the lifestyle (we have a full chapter on transitioning that begins on page 47), or you already eat this way yourself and are about to start a plant-based family. In these pages we meet you where you are and give you the tools and actionable advice you need to raise (and, more important, feed!) a happy and healthy plant-based family.

While we'd love to think that you might be so riveted by our words that you'll ignore everything going on in your life and simply sit down with this book until you've read every page, we know that you're busy and this isn't very likely. Thus, rather than reprising the research we presented in our last book, all of which demonstrates the myriad ways the Forks Over Knives lifestyle is the safest and healthiest diet there is, in this book we focus on only the most pertinent facts and applicable tips to help you implement the lifestyle in a busy family like yours. Our intention is that every time you pick up this book—whether it's for only five minutes or for longer—you will come away with something you can apply to your own life. So we present as much information as we can in as digestible a way as possible. To that end, there are a few regular features you'll find throughout the book to keep it fun and lively.

In each chapter, boxes titled **DID YOU KNOW?** present the most compelling facts about the medical benefits of this lifestyle in approachable, easy-to-grasp language. Our professional expertise is the underpinning of our ability to write authoritatively about nutrition and lifestyle, but our roles as Kylee and Jordan's parents inform a lot of this book. We are grateful for the opportunity writing this book gave us to channel fully all our knowledge and experience, be it medical or parental. However, as almost anyone will tell you, it is often important to differentiate between information that is rooted in professional expertise and enlightenment that comes from day-to-day life. So, periodically we share anecdotes that are unique to our particular experience as parents. We put these under the heading **OUR STORY** to signal that, to the extent possible, we've put aside our stethoscopes and are speaking as a mom and dad who are raising children in this lifestyle.

We are lucky that our working lives allow us to regularly see and hear all the different ways whole-food, plant-based eating can change people's lives for the better. When we decided to write this book, we knew we needed to find a way to share some of these real-life stories with our readers. So we asked the Forks Over Knives social media community to tell us about their experiences transitioning to and living in whole-food, plant-based families. The number of thoughtful and helpful responses we received touched and overwhelmed us. Thanks to the hundreds of people who took the time to write, we have many brief testimonials to share. These short **GETTING PERSONAL** accounts, which appear throughout the book, come from people at every stage of the plant-based journey, from those who are in the beginning months of their families' transitions to those who have been living plant-based for decades and raised their now-adult children this way.

Whether you're starting a family or are simply looking for ways to establish new habits in an already growing one, we've got you covered. But because every family is different and not every chapter may be relevant to your life, we list below the main topics covered in each. Note as well that the Contents (page vii) will guide you very quickly to each chapter. Whatever your personal circumstances, we hope the advice and tools we give and the stories we share will inspire you and put your family on a smooth path to a plant-based lifestyle.

Chapter 1: You're Having a Baby!

How to handle cravings and aversions. Finding a supportive doctor. Prenatal vitamins.

Chapter 2: Your Baby's First Year

What to eat while breastfeeding. When and how to introduce solids to baby.

Chapter 3: Beyond the First Year

Strategies to encourage good eating habits and discourage bad habits. Kids and supplements. Food sensitivities and allergies.

Chapter 4: How to Help Your Family Make the Forks Over Knives Transition

Hands-on approaches to changing your family's diet to a whole-food, plant-based one.

Chapter 5: Out of the House and on the Road

Handling social situations and celebrations, school lunches, traveling with kids.

Family Recipes

The second half of our book comprises valuable advice on plant-based cooking, as well as more than 125 delicious recipes for family-friendly meals, snacks, and desserts from Forks Over Knives Culinary Projects Manager Darshana Thacker.

PART I

THE FORKS OVER KNIVES FAMILY GUIDE

YOU'RE HAVING A BABY!

CHAPTER 1

Congratulations! You have embarked on one of the most profound and exciting journeys life has to offer. You likely have lots of questions and maybe a few concerns. Fundamental decisions that not that long ago were yours to make alone now have big implications for the little person growing inside you. It's no wonder that sometimes it can seem as if you're feeling joy and anxiety in equal measure. Thankfully, one thing does not have to be complicated: what and how much you should eat during pregnancy.

The Forks Over Knives guidelines for pregnant women are no different from those for anyone else. Eat whole, plant-based food—fruits, vegetables, tubers, whole grains, and legumes—until you are comfortably satiated. And when you are pregnant, eat as often as you need to in order to feel satisfied. If you're still transitioning to the Forks Over Knives lifestyle, this is a great time to take the leap and go fully whole-food, plant-based. Pregnancy is in some ways a delicate process, and it's important to be deliberate about your food choices. Foods that are harmful to you will be even more of a risk to the sensitive developing baby. The great news is that when you eat healthy, not only are you making the best choice for your baby but there are also some important benefits that you can look forward to for yourself. These benefits include a more appropriate weight gain; an easier time losing that weight after the baby

3

OUR STORY:
A Plant-Based Pregnancy Means More Energy

I certainly can't speak for every whole-food, plant-based mother ever, but based on my own pregnancies I can personally vouch for some pretty great benefits to this lifestyle. Not only did I experience everything listed on these pages, I also felt energetic all the way through both pregnancies. Sure, I was tired, but I was still able to do some form of exercise, such as walking, hiking, or using the elliptical machine every day until the time my water broke. After our second daughter, Jordan, was born, I could get up and go almost immediately. Jordan even joined her older sister, Kylee, at the park when she was only two days old! I'm pretty sure Jordan doesn't remember it, but I certainly do, and it was wonderful.

is delivered; minimal to no swelling in the face, hands, or legs; fewer skin issues (like acne or, paradoxically, excessive dryness); and best of all, a smoother delivery and faster recovery.

WHEN IS IT BEST TO BEGIN A WHOLE-FOOD, PLANT-BASED DIET?

Let's begin by saying that the best time to begin a whole-food, plant-based diet is always as soon as possible! That said, if you're a woman planning to get pregnant, ideally you want to make healthy changes beforehand. This will help ensure that your body is well nourished (and can begin eliminating environmental contaminants often concentrated in animal foods) for the organogenesis, or the formation of internal organs, that happens in the first ten to twelve weeks after conception, often before you even know you are pregnant. Furthermore, there are practical as well as emotional considerations that make it wise to transition pre-pregnancy, if possible. Getting your pantry and kitchen established as a whole-food, plant-based haven before you're pregnant means that you'll already know what foods you love. You'll also have a feel for how calorie density works, so if your caloric needs change or if pregnancy-induced aversions and cravings kick in, you'll have a deeper understanding and a broader plant-based repertoire to pull from to adapt and stay nourished. If your whole, plant-food habits are really well established, you'll even have some prepared food already stored in your freezer. This major convenience can be an absolute lifesaver when that first-trimester exhaustion hits!

On the other hand, though it's ideal to begin a whole-food, plant-based diet before you get pregnant, it's never too late to start. If you're far along in your pregnancy and you are ready to make the transition, go for it! Even changing just one meal a day is a great step. There is simply never a bad time to begin to improve your health, increase your vitality, and prevent disease.

There are as many different scenarios for what you may experience during your pregnancy as there are women in the world. It's not uncommon for the same woman to have multiple pregnancies that differ from one another significantly. You may have aversions or cravings; you might feel amazing or lousy— you might feel all of these things in a single week! Generally speaking, in the first trimester your appetite may be similar to what it was before you got pregnant. During the second and third trimesters, your appetite will increase, and you might eat more than usual. But you don't need to start counting calories! The beauty of the whole-food, plant-based lifestyle is the ability to listen to your hunger signals when they come calling. Better yet, when you address your hunger by eating good, healthy food, you won't have to worry about "getting all your nutrients." While every pregnancy is different no matter what Mom eats, the one thing that remains the same is that the whole-food, plant-based diet is the healthiest choice you can make for yourself and your baby.

CRAVINGS AND AVERSIONS

Just as our recommendation for what to eat is substantially the same whether or not you're pregnant, so is our advice for how to handle food-related impulses. Listen to your body and find ways to give it what it needs within the whole-food, plant-based model. If cravings have you focusing like a laser beam on a particular whole, plant-based food, go ahead and indulge. If it's a particularly calorie-dense food (see page xvi), don't worry about occasionally indulging in it unless you are keeping an eye on your weight because of health concerns. Whenever possible, add as many lower-calorie-density foods as you can to offset the higher-calorie-density foods.

If, on the other hand, your craving is for a food that is animal-based or highly processed, give your lifestyle a good look to make sure you're meeting your basic needs for ease and pleasure (see page xvi). Sometimes cravings for animal-based foods are more a sign of craving something easy, calorie-dense, or familiar. As such, there are often healthier, plant-based ways to meet those cravings. Once you confirm needs like ease and pleasure are being met, then you know your craving for food outside the whole-food, plant-based world is really about something else. We don't know exactly what causes cravings, but we do know that it's not an actual biological need for meat or dairy. So even when you seem unable to get those unhealthy foods out of your mind, remember that the cravings are not founded on a lack of a specific nutrient; more often it is a particular dish or flavor profile you are looking for (something sweet, salty, crunchy, hearty, etc.). Try to identify what it is about that food that you're craving, and then seek out healthier versions of that dish and flavor profile. For instance, if you can't stop thinking about a particular dairy-based sweet dessert, look for an alternative among the abundant whole-food, plant-based dessert options (you might want to begin with the Chocolate Sundae with Caramelized Bananas on page 257!).

When you are pregnant, it can be tempting, especially when you are faced with cravings, to really let loose and just eat anything you want. As we said previously, it's normal to eat somewhat more during pregnancy, but what you eat shouldn't be exclusively in the form of junk food. That can lead to big weight gains, which are not healthy for you or your baby. And you don't want to get into bad habits now that will be really hard to break a few months from now. As usual, planning in advance will help set you up for success. Make sure you have abundant healthy foods and snacks, including more calorie-dense ones, in the house, in the car, and at work to appease cravings. Also helpful is having on hand a supply of condiments that you love. For example, top a baked potato with a dip or dressing (check out the great recipes beginning on page 224); or stir nuts, seeds, or avocado into a bowlful of roasted vegetables to quickly satiate a yearning for something rich or creamy. The recipes for snacks beginning on page 106 provide some quick and easy solutions. Finally, it can be an enormous relief to have already prepared one or two of your favorite comfort foods, like mashed potatoes and gravy or brownies, to appease an acute craving when it hits.

Above all, don't ignore your cravings and hope they'll just go away! They are unlikely to vanish overnight, and you'll be far happier if you figure out how to satisfy them. On the other hand, don't let them rule you. Cravings come

OUR STORY:
Cravings and Aversions During Alona's Pregnancies

When I was pregnant, I had all sorts of cravings, but honestly they were no more frequent than usual. I *always* have cravings, especially for yummy sweets and desserts! I don't crave things outside of the whole-food, plant-based world, so I just did what I do when I'm not pregnant: when I wanted something badly enough, I went ahead and ate it. My bigger problems during my pregnancies were very strong aversions and extreme nausea and vomiting, coupled with a ravenous appetite. Not a comfortable combination! During the first trimester of both of my pregnancies I couldn't eat or even smell cooked vegetables, usually a major staple in my diet. I turned to raw vegetables like cucumbers and carrots, cauliflower dipped in hummus, and giant raw salads, but even there I struggled, because my aversions changed week to week, and sometimes even day to day. I remember one week in particular when tomatoes, which I'd been eating without issue for several weeks, suddenly became intolerable to me. Then, a few weeks later, I could suddenly enjoy them again. Perhaps worst of all, one of my absolute favorite desserts—a frozen banana with nut butter—was unbearable when I was pregnant. I couldn't *smell* a frozen banana without gagging.

Ultimately my only option was to eat small amounts of anything I could stomach throughout the day. My regular three daily meals were essentially replaced by a half dozen or more small snacks throughout the day. Since sour foods helped me stave off nausea, I began almost every morning with a chilled sour apple or lemon wedges. When I could eat salad, I'd make a big one at the beginning of the day and spoon out a little bit at different times all day long. When I couldn't tolerate salad, I turned to kidney beans and black beans, which worked for a while, as did fresh and frozen fruit for a time (except bananas, of course). I also tried to hide ingredients within a recipe. So, for example, I added spinach to my favorite carrot cake recipe or zucchini to a muffin recipe. I may not have been able to stomach these vegetables on their own, but tucking them into a dish where I couldn't really taste them was a great way to get veggies without gagging!

The most important thing I learned during my pregnancies was how necessary it was to really listen to my body, for there were usually only a few moments between my feeling hungry and becoming too nauseated to eat. This translated into sudden surges of hunger signaling that I needed to eat—*immediately*! I carried snacks wherever I went, usually in an insulated tote. This meant I always had with me an array of portable (and mostly durable) snacks that covered a range of calorie densities and that I could get excited about: carrots, apples, pears, raw cauliflower florets, berries, rice cakes, dried fruit, nuts, packaged LÄRABARS, and my favorite carrot cake. The bag didn't take long to pack up in the morning or night before. When hunger struck, I was able to rummage quickly and find at least one thing that I could tolerate.

Thank goodness Matt is a patient partner! More than once over the course of two pregnancies I asked him to pick up something at the store, only to be unable to eat it when he brought it home. In fact, he has a crucial bit of advice about cravings and aversions for the *partner* of anyone who is pregnant: be kind to your suddenly fickle partner! For some pregnant women, cravings can change on a dime. It's not unusual for a longing for an item to be as strong one day as the aversion to it is the day after. And take it from Matt—this is *not* the time to start lecturing your wife about eating her vegetables!

to all of us, whether or not we're pregnant. They may be more intense during pregnancy, but we always have the power to meet them within the whole-food, plant-based framework.

Aversions pose a different set of challenges. They can keep you from eating *enough* food. We hear a lot of statements like "I can't stand the smell of cooked broccoli." If this is the case for you, don't worry about eating the broccoli! People sometimes become fixated on having to "eat the rainbow" every day, but there is no need to think about your diet in such strict terms. Instead, over time, simply eat from each of the five categories—fruit, vegetables, tubers, whole grains, and legumes. If any given food within a category is nauseating to you, find something else that you can comfortably eat. For instance, if you're not loving mango, try an apple; if you just can't do collards, try carrots. Play around with more mild flavors: try potatoes, rice, or oil-free crackers. If you're having a very hard time keeping food down, it may become necessary to eat more calorie-dense foods so that you can get more caloric bang for your buck. Here's where avocado, nuts, nut butters, and dried fruits can help you. See Our Story on page 8 for specific details on how Alona handled her intense aversions during pregnancy. And if you're like Alona and having a nearly impossible time holding food down, focus on making every calorie count rather than on getting enough leafy greens. Indeed, it's more important in this situation to eat satisfying starchy foods such as sweet and white potatoes and grains like oats; leave the romaine salads for another day.

FINDING A SUPPORTIVE DOCTOR

If you've been plant-strong for years, it can be hard to discover that the very same doctor who was tolerant of that choice becomes unwilling to support your eating this way while pregnant. And if you're new to the whole-food, plant-based lifestyle, meeting this kind of opposition can be even more difficult. Unfortunately, when some people share with their obstetricians that they are whole-food, plant-based, the response is something along the lines of "Not anymore, you're not." This may be followed up by admonitions that there is no way a pregnant woman can eat this diet and consume sufficient calcium, protein, iron, and every other nutrient a healthy baby needs. This is a fallacy. When you eat a whole-food, plant-based diet, not only do you get just what you need from your food (as we talk about on page xii), but you also get it in a package that doesn't have harmful side effects for you *and* your baby.

Hold tight to the conviction that you are making the best possible choice for you and your baby, and have sufficient confidence in this decision to keep looking until you find a doctor who will support your choice. Remember that a supportive doctor does not have to live or actively promote a whole-food, plant-based lifestyle him- or herself (although, naturally, in an ideal world that would always be the case everywhere). A supportive doctor needs to be open-minded and willing to support *your* choices for you and your family.

If your doctor expresses skepticism about your diet, you may need to help him or her along by sharing information. Don't be surprised! Most doctors are not trained in nutrition, so they may not be any more knowledgeable than any-one else about which foods are best for you and your baby. Many doctors can move fairly quickly from resistance to support once they recognize that you choose to eat this way based on knowledge. It can help just to talk to them. There is no litmus test for finding a supportive and caring doctor, and this is no doubt one of a handful or more issues that you'll want to discuss anyway. Simply add it to your list of questions, and if you get the feeling that he or she is going to be dogmatic about *anything* in a way that doesn't sit right with you, look for another doctor.

And while we're on the topic of doctors, pregnancy is often the time when expectant parents begin the search for a pediatrician for their children. We are often asked for advice on how to find one who supports the whole-food, plant-based lifestyle. Our answer here is very similar to our advice for finding a doctor for yourself during pregnancy: it is more beneficial to find a doctor

---

DID YOU KNOW? When you eat a whole-food, plant-based diet, 75 to 80 percent of your calories will come from carbohydrates—and that is precisely what you want. The unrefined carbs in whole and minimally processed plant foods do not cause diabetes or make us fat. In fact, studies show that the lowest rates of diabetes in the world are found among populations that consume the most carbohydrates.[4]

---

who is open to and accommodating of your dietary choices, even if that doctor isn't a vocal proponent of whole-food, plant-based living. Focus instead on finding someone who is thoughtful and sensitive, who listens to you, and who will respect your healthy lifestyle choices, even if he or she does not live and eat the same way. There is more to each doctor's visit than discussions about your child's diet, and it's as important that you feel comfortable with the pediatrician's views on all the issues you care about, as it is that he or she is open to your food choices. As long as your child is healthy and growing, a pediatrician is unlikely to press you on your family's diet. It is when a child is struggling that there is more room for disagreement. This is when it's especially important that you have a doctor who is willing to work with you within your whole-food, plant-based preferences.

PRENATAL VITAMINS: SHOULD YOU TAKE THEM OR LEAVE THEM?

Women often wonder whether they need to take vitamins during pregnancy, even if they don't take them ordinarily. As we said earlier, all whole, plant-based foods contain carbohydrates, protein, and fat, as well as almost every vitamin and mineral the human body needs, so there is generally not a need to take supplements (with the exception of B_{12}; see page 43). This doesn't change when you are pregnant. Just eat a generous amount of vegetables and other whole, plant-based foods, and your body will extract what it needs from the nourishing foods that you consume.

There's a faulty perception in America that we are somehow deficient by nature and that consuming more nutrients, even in pill form, is always better. In reality the Standard American Diet is over-indulgent and under-nutritious. Over the last century, the quality of the American diet deteriorated precipitously. That led to deficiencies across the population, which is a significant reason we see to-day's nearly ubiquitous prescribing of prenatal vitamins for women who are even thinking about wanting to get pregnant.

If that comes as a surprise, it's because we've been inundated by main-stream dogma about pregnancy and nutrition, which treats nutrients as a problem to be solved, hand-in-hand with the philosophy that "more is better" (You're deficient! This pill is your answer!), rather than regarding nutrients simply as what is contained in the nourishing package of whole, plant-based food. But the ironic truth is that throughout history, deficiencies—and some-times the diseases caused by them—came about as people began "improving" natural foods. For instance, when rice polishing, wherein the outer, thiamine-rich husk is removed from each grain to make it less susceptible to spoil-age, became widespread in Asia, a very real disease—Beriberi—caused by thiamine-deficiency also became prevalent.[5]

Certainly there are nutrients such as folate and iron that are especially important for baby and mother alike during pregnancy. But regular supple-mentation of synthetic folic acid didn't become widespread until we lost access to naturally occurring folate—a B vitamin abundant in many plant foods—largely because we started eating fewer plants and foliage and consum-ing more refined and processed foods. Folate is important during pregnancy, especially during the first few weeks, for the healthy growth of your baby's spinal cord and brain. You may be more familiar with folic acid, because the terms "folate" and "folic acid" are used almost interchangeably in our lan-guage. But the substances definitely are *not* interchangeable. There are known risks associated with synthetic folic acid; it is associated with increased cancer risk and all-cause mortality.[6] There are *no* risks associated with natural folate from food.

The primary cause of nutritional deficiency for most people is that they don't eat nearly enough fruits, vegetables, tubers, whole grains, and legumes to meet their needs. For people eating the Standard American Diet, which combines a dearth of nutrient-rich vegetables with an abundance of foods that can actually interfere with nutrient absorption, such as dairy, specific supplementation of these highly important nutrients is likely wise. But our advice is to get your nutrition from your food, which is superior to getting it from supplements. When people eat a healthy whole-food, plant-based diet, as defined on page xi, they will get the nutrients they need, and in general will not require additional supplements, even during pregnancy.

The real issue is that if you're eating an unhealthy diet, you are more likely to have deficiencies; in that case, is taking a supplement better than not taking one? The answer is that we really don't know. There is evidence that supplements will help (folic acid supplements reduce the risk of neural tube defects), but they come with potential harm (supplemental folic acid increases the risk of breast cancer by 20 to 30 percent). On the other hand, 2,000 calories, or a day's worth for most people, comprising one food from each of the five categories of a healthy whole-food, plant-based diet (about 1 pound each of mangoes, cooked spinach, sweet potato, brown rice, and white beans) will give you 1,270 micrograms of folate, or 318 percent of the recommended daily allowance. That's all the folate you need without any of the side effects or potential harm from folic acid.

Ultimately, our advice is to consult with your doctor to rule in or out a deficiency. If you are not deficient, then whether or not you should take prenatal vitamins depends on your consultation with your doctor, your comfort level, and how healthful your diet is. If you decide to take supplements, we recommend to our patients that they avoid those catchalls that are jam-packed with lots of extras you don't need. It is especially important to avoid any that contain large concentrations of nutrients that have been shown to be harmful when consumed as part of a supplement (such as vitamins A, E, and beta-carotene).[7] No matter what you choose as far as supplementation, your first focus should always be on trying to meet your needs naturally with food. Deficiencies are much more likely to be an issue if you're not eating well. So eat well!

DID YOU KNOW? Minerals like calcium, iron, magnesium, and copper are found in the soil, where they are absorbed into the roots of plants. Animals get their minerals when they eat the plants that absorb them. This means that the animals many consider to be good sources of minerals actually get them secondhand from plants, and so should we.

OUR STORY: Alona's Nutritional Bank

I adopted a whole-food, plant-based diet after extensive research. Matt and I have been eating and living this way for many years, and I know personally how healthy and vibrant it makes me feel. I am a trained doctor who specializes in nutrition and lifestyle medicine, and I have seen firsthand the evidence of the lifestyle's extensive benefits. In short, in both my personal and my professional life, I am a champion for the whole-food, plant-based lifestyle.

But pregnancy is an emotional time. Sure, I knew in my head that I very likely didn't *need* to go out of my way to eat specific foods for their nutrients. For instance, I knew absolutely that I was getting enough folate from what I was eating. But my emotional heart needed insurance. I thought about it hard and did my own analysis of whatever perceived risk I was trying to mitigate compared to the risk of taking a supplement. That's when I began to think of my diet as a "nutritional bank" into which I could deposit extra amounts of specific foods for nutritional insurance. When I'm not pregnant, I don't consider it a big deal if I don't eat perfectly every single day. When I was pregnant, though, it felt more important to eat very deliberately. Once I'd determined that I wasn't going to take any supplemental vitamins as long as my blood work came back in healthy ranges, I focused on the foods that I knew were important.

So, to supply that nutritional bank and reassure myself, I made sure I had extra helpings of folate-rich greens and legumes, as well as cooked soybeans, white beans, lentils, and spinach for iron. I added an extra tablespoon of chia seeds or ground flaxseed in my food every day for concentrated sources of omega-3 fatty acids. Ultimately, I had two healthy, supplement-free pregnancies—and a peaceful heart.

GETTING PERSONAL

When I have morning sickness, it can be hard to eat greens, so I just blend them up in a fruit smoothie to get them in, and it is delicious! I have also enjoyed eating until I feel satisfied without feeling any regrets. There is nothing better than knowing that you are giving your baby the best start in life by eating a plant-based diet during pregnancy.
—Jennifer Beh, Ogden, Utah; five children, ages 3 months, 2, 4, 6, and 8

I read a few books about vegan pregnancy, but I found myself worrying over my protein and vitamin intake so much that it was seriously stressing me out. I ended up ditching the "textbook" regime and I went back to eating what made me feel good. A few times, I had people, some complete strangers, express concern for my and my baby's well-being, but I simply thanked them for their concern and assured them that I knew what was right for my and my baby's bodies. My OB was thrilled with my diet. I remember him asking if I planned to stay vegan the whole pregnancy and then sighing with relief when I said yes.
—Jessica White-Cason, Las Cruces, New Mexico; one child, age 1

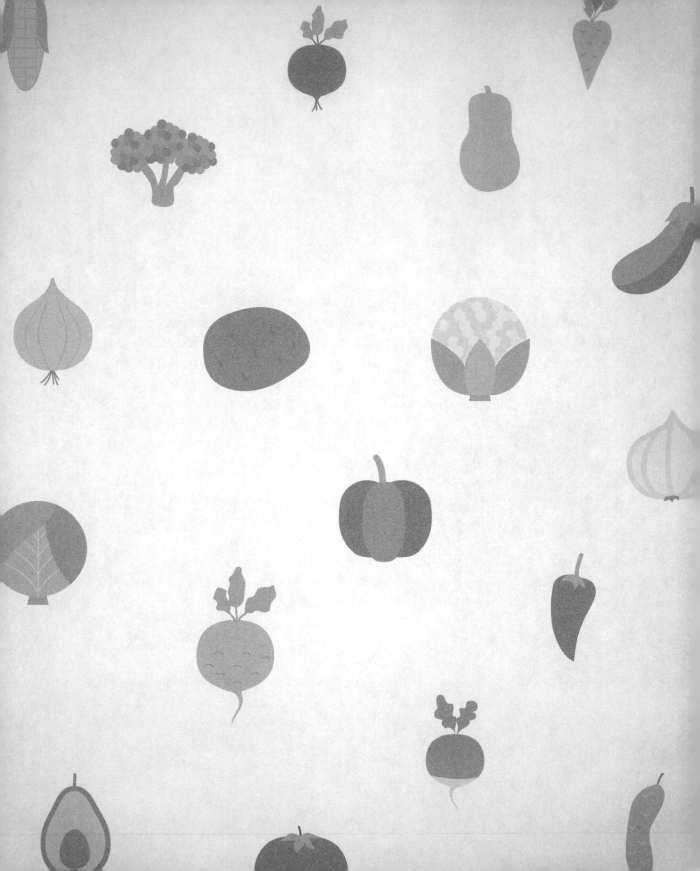

CHAPTER 2

YOUR BABY'S FIRST YEAR

The first year of life is a time of extraordinary change and growth. In a mere twelve months your new little person will transform from a tiny eating-and-pooping machine to a bundle of energy who crawls or toddles faster than you can believe. It's good to keep this in mind when feeding your baby this year. If some stages seem challenging, remember none of them last more than a few months!

From the start, we recommend breastfeeding as long as you possibly can: at least six months if possible and ideally a year or more. The longer you can breastfeed during your baby's first year, the healthier it is for your baby, and for you. If breastfeeding is not possible, there are alternative options, such as pumping your breast milk or buying from a breast milk bank and offering it in a bottle. If these options are not feasible, there are infant formulas that are aligned with a plant-based diet. Talk to your child's pediatrician about options that might work for you and your baby.

While you are breastfeeding, you can continue to eat the same whole, plant-based foods that you've enjoyed all along, with one caveat. Avoid any foods your baby appears to be sensitive to. For example, steer clear of eating cabbage if you find that every time you eat it your baby gets gassy or unusually fussy after nursing. Note there may also be a delay between when you eat a particular food and your baby's negative reaction to it, so look back two or more meals if the most immediate meal doesn't provide any answers to consistent fussiness after nursing. Babies sometimes just get fussy, so only be concerned about this if you see a consistent pattern after multiple meals. No matter what you eliminate from your diet, there are always many other plant-based foods available to you. Breastfeeding consumes calories, so you may be hungry a little more frequently than usual (much like during pregnancy). Just eat when you are hungry and until comfortably satiated. Don't worry about controlling your intake in order to lose the "baby weight" during this period (it may affect milk production if you do). When you eat a whole-food, plant-based diet, you can feel fine about eating when you're hungry, and there is even compelling anecdotal evidence that breastfeeding women return to their pre-baby weight more quickly than those who don't breastfeed.

INTRODUCING SOLIDS

In most cases, babies need only breast milk for the first five or six months of their lives, after which time you can begin to introduce some solids while you continue to breastfeed (which, again, we urge you to continue for as long as is feasible). Some babies consume only breast milk even longer. In fact, we regard weaning as a process that can last anywhere from about six months to several years. Your child will often let you know when she is ready to try some "real" food. Introduce solids when your baby is showing signs of interest. Watch her body language for cues. Is she watching your fork as it moves from plate to mouth? Is she reaching for your fork or your plate? Does she seem more interested in what's going on at your place at the table than what is in front of her? These are all good signs that she's ready to begin.

The first thing many parents look to add to a baby's diet when beginning to wean is a dairy-based alternative to breast milk, but this is unnecessary. Children don't need to drink milk *of any kind* after weaning. If at five months or so it seems that your baby is hungry for something more than breast milk but is not yet ready for solids, we recommend preparing a homemade mixture that can be put in a bottle. We used a good one that's based on sweet potato puree: simply mix a few spoonfuls of pureed sweet potato with water. Some parents we have worked with choose to add a little unsweetened soymilk. If you decide to go that route, we recommend adding just a small amount and using a brand that lists only soybeans and water in the ingredients (we use the organic unsweetened plain version made by Westsoy). The other nondairy milks tend to have unhealthier ingredients like added sodium, sugar, supplements, thickeners, and flavors, so we recommend avoiding those. And remember that water should ideally be the primary liquid used. For the puree, you can use either jarred baby food or homemade; just make sure that it is very smooth and sufficiently diluted so that it won't block the bottle nipple. Also, be sure to use the nipples with larger openings for this mixture. As our babies got older and wanted to keep their bottles, we had to actually cut the holes in the nipples bigger. They essentially were eating sweet potato puree but preferred getting it from the bottle rather than the spoon. Don't worry; they will eventually give up the bottles. Our preference is to allow the child to gauge what she wants when it involves things that don't really impact her health.

If your baby is at least six months old and you are ready for some separation, but she is not giving any signs that she's ready to explore foods in addition to breast milk, it might be time to be intentional. Begin by breastfeeding a little less frequently. Find the time during the day when your baby needs to breastfeed the least—usually sometime in the middle of her busy day—and offer a bottle with an alternative such as the sweet-potato-based mixture just mentioned. (Or, if she's old enough to wean but hasn't ever adopted a bottle, just skip the bottle and go straight to a sippy cup.)

When you first introduce solid foods, she may only begin with a bite or two. This is fine; over time she'll certainly want more. If she seems very resistant, try giving her a little breast milk before again offering her the solid food. Paradoxically, a very hungry baby is often not receptive to solid food, which she won't yet associate with making the hunger go away. But once those hunger pangs have lessened thanks to the breast milk, she's more likely to be ready to investigate unfamiliar foods. The key to success is to keep trying and remember this is a partnership between you and your child. If you are feeling tired of breastfeeding, but your child wants to continue, try to find a compromise in the middle. All too often, parents focus on their child's needs at the expense of their own, which can teach the child that her parents' needs don't matter as much as her own do.

Adding solids to your baby's diet does not in any way have to mean that she'll hop on the fast track right off of breastfeeding. Babies tend to eat very little when first starting on solid foods, and it takes several months for them to eat enough to wholly take the place of breast milk. They still need that nourishment, which is one of the reasons we urge giving babies breast milk until they are at least one year old. And as we said previously, weaning from an all-breast-milk diet to an all-solid diet can take from months to years, depending on your and your baby's needs and preferences.

FEEDING BABY SOLIDS: WHAT FOODS TO START WITH

We don't believe in hard-and-fast rules for what order to introduce solids to your baby (see Our Story, page 26, for how we did it). Unless your child shows a sensitivity to a particular food, the only plant-based foods that we recommend avoiding for the first year are nuts (choking hazard); strawberries, because some children show allergies to them when they are introduced too early; and if choosing to include nondairy milks, then avoid those that include anything other than the main ingredient (i.e., soybeans or almonds) and water (see

DID YOU KNOW? There is a connection between dairy and type 1 diabetes. Studies have shown that the immune system sometimes struggles to differentiate between the amino acids in dairy and insulin-producing cells in our pancreas that look identical (they have similar amino acid chains). This means that when some babies consume dairy products, their immune system attacks not only the dairy proteins in the blood but also the similar-looking proteins (amino acid chains) in the pancreas, which can result in so much damage to the pancreatic cells that they no longer produce insulin. The result is type 1 diabetes. In fact, one study showed that the risk of developing type 1 diabetes is more than five times greater in people who consume three or more glasses of milk per day.[8] Kids who give up dairy tend to have fewer ear infections and thus less need for antibiotics, as well as fewer colds and less mucous production. There is a strong connection between dairy and constipation, as well as a link between dairy and acne in children.[9] Dairy is also a common cause of food allergies, especially in children, and there is a possible link between dairy consumption and asthma risk or lung reactivity. Many people see certain symptoms resolve or lessen very quickly once all dairy is removed from the diet.[10]

page 21). We also don't recommend drinking juices or nondairy milks alone by the glass or bottle.*

---

* Strictly speaking, honey is not a plant-based food, but we know that some plant-based eaters include it in their diets. Thus we are compelled to add that babies under the age of 1 should not consume honey. It contains spores of *Clostridium botulinum* bacteria, which older children and adults can easily digest. The immature digestive systems of very young children cannot handle them, however, and ingesting these bacteria can lead to botulism, impairing a baby's ability to feed, move, or breathe.

Our suggestion is to introduce just one new food to your baby each day and do it in the morning rather than later in the day. This way if he has any reaction, you'll know it's probably to the new food and you or your baby's caretaker can see it while the baby is up, instead of the baby having the reaction overnight while sleeping. (For more on food sensitivities and allergies, see page 45.)

Don't assume that your child will love everything you introduce the first time he tastes it; nor that if he spits it out the first few times you offer it, he'll never learn to like it. Kids can certainly have natural aversions to particular foods, as can adults, but this does not mean that when you try to serve him green beans three different times and he rejects it each time it's because he'll *never* like green beans. We have found that in some cases it can take as many as ten or more separate encounters with a particular food over several months before a child might learn to like it. (One of Kylee's favorite foods is collard greens; this is likely because she is regularly exposed to them and not because she was somehow inherently drawn to them.) Also, keep in mind that kids are fickle. One day they won't eat something and the next they'll eat a whole bowl of it. The key is to keep trying and be creative! We find that playing games with our children helps improve consumption. For example, Kylee loves to play "guess what that was": we have her close her eyes and then put something (usually a vegetable) on a spoon and put it in her mouth. She tries to name what she just ate. Occasionally we will sneak in a chocolate nut-butter truffle just to keep her interested and engaged, hoping that one of the bites may be the special treat. For her part, Jordan likes when we take a special Disney princess plate and cover it with food (we usually save this for vegetables, too). Then she tries to eat away all the food to reveal the different princesses.

Sometimes it helps to combine new foods you're introducing with their favorites. If your baby loves sweet potatoes, for example, try mixing some greens or peas into them. This way he still has that familiar, desirable flavor and texture, but he also tastes a new food. Or, if he doesn't like a particular food in one form, try serving it another way. So if mashed green beans are not going down easy, turn them into finger foods by cutting them into small pieces. Just make

---

DID YOU KNOW? How much calcium you get isn't as important as where you get it. A diet high in animal products, even when high in calcium, is actually associated with worse bone health. That's right: populations with higher calcium consumption (usually from dairy products) tend to have higher fracture rates.[11] Eating a whole-food, plant-based diet gives your body the calcium and other nutrients it needs for healthy bones.

---

sure to cook them until they are soft enough that they can be squished without teeth. We also like to hide the beans under the mashed potatoes and then the girls try to eat down and find the hidden "treasure."

Kids have strong preferences and they don't necessarily love variety, often preferring the same tried-and-true dishes over your innovations. We know from experience how frustrating it is to spend an hour preparing a meal only to have it fall on "deaf" mouths. All too often when Jordan sees a new dish coming, she will start yelling "I don't like it" before it has gotten close enough for her to smell, let alone taste, it! Most kids' palates prefer food blander than adults' do. If there are things that he likes, these will become the staples that he eats. If it happens to be the same thing every day for a while, or if he doesn't eat much for a day or so, don't worry. On the other hand, if you suspect that his decrease in eating might be boredom with a food you've offered regularly, substitute something else. Thankfully there are so many choices in the whole-food, plant-based universe that it is easy to avoid getting into a rut.

Finally, once you've introduced a few different items, don't feel compelled to prepare food for your baby that is completely different from what you're cooking for the rest of the family. Just go ahead and offer what you're eating to baby. Short of the few exceptions we mentioned in this chapter, there is very little you can't introduce to him in his first year.

OUR STORY:
Kylee's and Jordan's Self-Serve Eating

We did not follow an intricate schedule for introducing solids to Kylee and Jordan. We began by offering fruits like apples, pears, and bananas, as well as squashes, yams, potatoes, and carrots. After that it depended on what they liked. Some people prefer to start with vegetables before they introduce fruits because they are nervous that once babies taste sweet fruit, they'll never eat a vegetable. We didn't find that to be a problem. Our kids love any kind of fruit and also happily eat vegetables like kale, broccoli, and collard greens, so we didn't encounter this challenge at all.

A bigger challenge for us than what they'd eat is whether they'd slow down long enough to eat at all. Neither of them had much patience for sitting still for a meal. So, we came up with healthy drinks. For Kylee we made a drink mixture of pureed cooked collards, sweet potatoes, and oat milk. For Jordan we began with a simple mixture of pureed sweet potatoes and water (described in detail on page 21).

As they grew and we introduced more foods, we tried to be intentional about their options. Don't get us wrong. They certainly get treats, but they don't eat a lot of junk food. To satisfy their innate preference for sweets, we've just always focused on naturally sweet foods. Since these are the sorts of foods they are offered most often, this kind of eating is their habit. Once a kid has tasted Cheetos, it's going to be more of a struggle to get her to eat even fruit, because its natural sweetness and delectability pales in comparison to artificially sweetened, salty, high-fat foods. This is the Dopamine Pleasure Cycle we talked about in the Introduction. The more of these hyper-stimulating foods a person eats (no matter their age), the more the body craves them and the less satisfying healthy foods are by comparison. So, during these early days be mindful of the choices you make for your child. The practices and foods you introduce to them now, when they are learning about eating and taste for the very first time, are fundamental to how they will perceive food for the rest of their lives; try to be sure you're making the healthiest choices you can.

Over time we've established which habits and foods work best for our girls (many of their favorites are listed on page 32). We have a lower shelf in the refrigerator dedicated to holding only their snacks. They can help themselves when they are hungry, which is very important for a child. Allowing even young children to have control over their own hunger is crucial for their physical *and* emotional growth. We don't generally fret about whether they'll "ruin" their dinner. When what you're offering is good for them, you won't need to say that. Furthermore, for us, dinner is a time of gathering for the family that is not optional, but how much people eat is up to them. Instead of monitoring their every bite at the dinner table, we can instead focus on enjoying our time together.

GETTING PERSONAL

Since we were already following a vegan diet, we didn't have to worry about eliminating animal products. However, it's been a bigger challenge to eliminate vegan junk food from our lives. One challenge we've had is trying to get our son to ask for fewer unhealthy vegan foods, such as processed vegan cheeses and vegan soy products. One way we've overcome that challenge is to keep all those foods out of our home and only serve whole, plant-based foods. We also limit the number of unhealthy foods he can eat when he is at an event where vegan junk food is served. The better example that I set, the less my son asks for the types of food I'd like him to avoid eating.

—Andrea Zollman, Los Angeles, California; one child, age 11

My son is an extremely picky eater, but I've found that this is the easiest way to feed him. He loves fruit, some vegetables, wheat bread, and baked goods. It's been really easy to make whole-food, plant-based items like muffins and pancakes, but he has no idea that they're healthy so he doesn't feel like he's giving anything up. And the dishes I make for dinner consist of a lot of his favorite ingredients. He doesn't often eat them in their entirety, but if I take out ingredients (say, set aside some sweet potatoes and peas for him before they go into the curry), then he happily eats.

—Lindsay Maxfield, Salt Lake City, Utah; three children, ages 5 and 2 (twins)

Parents do not need to be so food fixated when it comes to children. Feed them a wide variety of whole plant foods and relax. Have fun. Don't stress! KEEP IT SIMPLE! Eat foods in as natural a state as possible to reduce time spent worrying and preparing. Invest in good tools! I can't live without my Vitamix, Bosch Universal machine, grain mill, food chopper, food processor, and some quality knives and cookware!

—Lisa Gladden-Kuettle, Bend, Oregon; five adult children

CHAPTER 3

BEYOND THE FIRST YEAR

When your child reaches her first birthday, she'll be ready to eat pretty much anything you eat. At this time you may find yourself swayed by the predominant message coming from the USDA and other sources that every day's meals should be a specific balance of dairy, "protein," grains, vegetables, and fruit. But we're here to reassure you that you don't have to think about what you feed your children in terms of precise amounts of specific categories of foods. Over the course of a week you simply need to offer your child these whole foods: fruits, vegetables, tubers, whole grains, and legumes. You don't have to select foods in order to target specific nutrients (like protein). Further, don't fret that you must always serve food in entirely composed meals that fit the conventional ideas of "breakfast, lunch, and dinner." Just have these foods available and be sure your meals are built around starches and fruits, as discussed on page xi. Feed your kids what they love. Does your kid like lasagna? It makes a great breakfast. And pancakes are a favorite dinner for lots of families.

DID YOU KNOW? Dietary fiber satisfies the hunger drive and binds to and assists in the elimination of excess hormones, toxins, cholesterol, and other undesirable matter. Foods naturally high in fiber also help stabilize blood sugar. Consuming a significant number of calories that don't have fiber will significantly increase the risk of constipation because the bowel requires fiber to function properly. Whole, unrefined plant foods are the best sources of dietary fiber. Animal-based and refined, processed foods do not contain fiber.

IS MY CHILD EATING THE RIGHT AMOUNT OF FOOD?

We see two contrasting worries come up when parents feed their kids a whole-food, plant-based diet: one, that they're eating enormous amounts of food; or, two, that they're not eating enough. In fact, there is no "right" amount to feed a child when he is eating a whole-food, plant-based diet. To a larger extent than most adults, the volume kids eat day to day will fluctuate. They will go some days with little intake and other days with significantly more.

So, don't be surprised if he eats much more food than his omnivore friends. The reason for this is simple: plant foods are less calorie dense; that is, they have fewer calories per bite of food, so a plant-eating child will eat more volume to reach satiation and an adequate amount of calories. On the other hand, if your child seems more interested in playing than in eating, it is equally no cause for alarm. Sometimes it feels like Kylee and Jordan go days almost eating nothing at all and then all of a sudden they put their parents to shame, eating so much that we check the floor to be sure they really did consume everything. There are many perfectly ordinary reasons for a child's temporarily lower intake. It could be because he ate enough or too much at the few meals prior, so he's balancing out now; or he has a little virus, and eating less is actually protective (it allows the body to focus energy on fighting infection rather than on digestion); or he's teething and it hurts to eat. Most often this is temporary and rarely a sign of something significant. As we've said previously, many pediatricians say it is not what a kid eats in a day but what he eats in a *week* that counts.

In short, generally you can trust that kids will get enough food by eating when they are hungry. As hard as it can seem sometimes, simply continue to trust your child's internal signals, and make healthy food options available throughout the day. In our experience, it's generally not a good idea to "push" kids to eat, not least because it rarely results in their eating much more. For the often hard-won advantage of getting a few extra bites in them (at most), you can cause a lot of anxiety for both you and your child, and those few small bites do little to improve his overall nutritional status. His hunger signals, or lack of hunger signals, will prevail over even the most anxious parents.

When we worry about our children's consumption it's because we're concerned that they're not getting sufficient nutrition. The truth is that there's no definitive way to know exactly how many calories and nutrients—carbohydrates, essential fats, essential amino acids, vitamins, and minerals—children need to eat daily to thrive. Moreover, the actual amounts needed likely fluctuate from day to day and the gastrointestinal tract can increase or decrease absorption of nutrients when we are off by a little bit. It's much more valuable to focus on good-tasting whole, plant-based foods than to worry about the specific nutrients; these things take care of themselves when we're making the right food choices.

We also know that the best way to ensure adequate nutrient consumption is to trust your child's hunger signals, and make sure every calorie counts. The more healthy foods he eats, the less room there is for the unhealthy ones—it's as if the good stuff crowds out the lousy junk. It's also wise to avoid sweeteners, oils, and other highly processed foods. These foods can meet a body's caloric needs, but do so without providing sufficient nutrients. So, the more unhealthy foods a child consumes, the less you can trust that his nutrient needs are being met based on hunger signals alone.

KID-FRIENDLY SNACKS

Frankly, far more important than concerns about what constitutes a proper meal is that your kids enjoy eating the food that's available in the house—so that they'll eat it! Here are some kid-friendly favorites that make great snacks or anytime food:

- Cut-up fresh fruit, especially melon. (In our house, Alona often cuts up a bunch of fruit in the morning for her own breakfast and then leaves behind containers in the fridge for the girls to have during the day.)

- Baby carrots with hummus.

- Frozen bananas, mangoes, and blueberries.

- Oil-free crackers (corn thins, brown rice or seaweed crackers) with bean dip.

- Steamed rice stirred into lentil dip.

- Brown rice cakes with avocado or nut butter.

- Rinsed and drained chickpeas (these are great finger foods).

- Pureed fruit-and-vegetable mixtures in pouches and jarred baby food.

- Nuts and seeds (after the age of 1).

- Baked, oil-free corn chips and guacamole.

- Little containers of applesauce.

- LÄRABARS.

- Dried fruit.

- Fruit ice "creams" (see page 258).

OUR STORY:
The Impulse to "Push" Food

Given all the "don't push food" advice we dispense on these pages, you might assume that we'd be entirely unruffled by our girls' variable appetites and periodic food strikes.

Actually, the opposite is true. In our roles as doctors advising other families, it's second nature to us to think logically. With our own family, however, we also sometimes think emotionally. Occasionally we catch ourselves pushing food on the girls, especially Kylee, our very active older daughter. This does little more than relieve our own worry while adding to her level of anxiety. Our girls continue to grow and thrive. This is just one of many times as parents we have to manage our own angst rather than try to persuade our perfectly healthy children to do anything differently.

So, when Kylee just can't be bothered to slow down and eat, we provide more of her favorite, easy-to-grab food such as dried fruits and nuts for her snacks that day. Sometimes she finds smaller portions less overwhelming, so we also freeze small amounts of foods—purees and combinations of chopped fruit and steamed vegetables—in ice cube trays. Then we can defrost just a small amount for a busy kid a few times a day rather than a full plate that she'll never finish.

Jordan loves to wash dishes, so she tends to eat her food and "clean her plate" when we let her do the dishes afterwards. Given she is 2 years old, rarely does this actually help us in any way other than getting her excited to finish the food on her dish before she is allowed to clean it. At the end of the day, we find that little tricks like these, which indirectly encourage eating, are far more successful than more overtly pushing food.

STRATEGIES TO ENCOURAGE GOOD EATING

The best way to inspire kids to eat more good food is to get them involved and engaged before anyone is even sitting at the dinner table. It's wise to show them that food doesn't come out of a box; it comes from the earth. And teaching your kids how to *prepare* healthy food—and really letting them get their hands (and your kitchen) dirty—is the key to teaching them to *eat* healthy food. Here are some specific approaches to get them on board.

Let the kids loose in the kitchen. We've seen this implemented in many different ways; there's certainly no one, "right" way to do it. One we like is to let your child choose a dish for the family's dinner. Depending on your child's age, how many other children you have, and how many plant-based dishes your kids are familiar with, she can choose one dish for every night's dinner or just one dish during the week. For older kids, it can mean that you let them pick *and* prepare the dish (with your help, at least at first). For younger kids, you can offer them a choice of two or three dishes or recipes from which they can choose one. Then ask them to help you prepare it. Kids of almost any age can be helpful—or at least can believe they're being helpful. Toddlers and preschoolers can clean vegetables, add ingredients to bowls, and toss salads. Elementary school–age kids can use a small paring knife to trim vegetables, measure ingredients, and even stir things in pans with supervision. Older tweens and teens can take on and prepare by themselves an entire dish—and, eventually, a whole meal. Try not to focus on the mess they'll surely make. Remember, they won't always be under your roof. You're not only getting them interested and invested in what they're eating, you're teaching them valuable life skills.

Begin with dessert. As a corollary to the point above, some parents report success when they ask their kids to make dessert—whole-food, plant-based dessert, of course! Sometimes knowing what they have to look forward to, and the pride of having made it themselves, can motivate a kid to eat what Mom or Dad prepared for the main course.

Show them how it grows. Spark an interest in eating by pulling back the curtain on how and where food grows. Take your kids to a farmers' market or to a farm—berry- and apple-picking excursions are great for both fun and enlightenment. If possible, grow some of your own food. It can be as simple as a pot of herbs on a porch, patio, or in a sunny window or as involved as a backyard plot with vegetables, fruit, and herbs. Put their natural affinity for getting dirty to good use with planting seeds, pruning seedlings, and, if you're lucky, doing a little weeding. Offer them some of their "own" plants, and, most important, let them harvest the bounty when it's ready.

Make it a game. Suggest an "experiment" for the whole family: You all agree to incorporate one new fruit or vegetable into your dinner every week; make it one you currently don't prepare ever or very often. Have the kids participate in choosing how the new item will be served—raw or cooked, plain or with sauce, on its own or hidden in a dish. Emphasize that no one has to like everything; you all agree merely to try it. Keep a running list of what you've tried and how it was prepared and whether the group generally liked or did not like it. The refrigerator is a favorite spot for this list in many households, so that the whole family can keep track of its shared progress. The keys here are that everyone should be willingly involved and that there is no judgment or pressure. You want to avoid telling your kids that they *must* eat this or that. To encourage really young kids, fun plates or placemats with pictures on them—trucks, dinosaurs, animals, princesses, maps of the United States, the list is endless—can become a canvas that they "unpaint." Strategically place small amounts of food over a few different areas of the image and challenge them to reveal what's underneath.

Take the taste test challenge. Set up a taste test of a single ingredient presented two or three different ways. Everyone can try them all and decide how they like them. For example, carrots can be shredded in a salad with raisins and nuts, sliced into sticks and served with dipping sauce, or cut into coins and stir-fried. Garbanzo beans can be placed in a salad, ground up to make hummus and spread into a sandwich, or toasted and enjoyed on their own as a crispy snack. With younger kids sometimes you don't even need to change the flavor profile because changing the shape is enough to make them think it's a taste test. We sometimes switch up the usual microwave-steamed potato rounds we serve Kylee and instead slice the potatoes lengthwise into long sticks or wedges. We cook them the same way but call them "fries" and all at once she and Jordan think they're something completely different and wonderful!

Use your hands! Many kids we know are much more enthusiastic about eating when they are freed from the "rigid" constraints of proper dining etiquette. Put another way, they just really like to eat with their hands. There is a large selection of kid-friendly dipping sauces beginning on page 224. Keep the forks in the drawer for a night and try a "dipping dinner" at which you serve two or three dipping sauces with a few dippable foods. Plus, there's no law that we know of that states soup has to be served with a spoon. Bell pepper wedges and sliced whole-grain bread are excellent ways to get thick soups from bowl to mouth. Pureed soup can double as a dipping sauce for "fries" or veggies.

HALFWAY THERE AND STUCK FAST: GETTING OUT OF A RUT

Some parents report that their children will happily eat the whole, plant-based food they prepare. The problem is with the variety: he'll only eat two dishes! Here the challenge is to expand the repertoire, and, here again, making a game of it is often the best approach.

For kids with any degree of reluctance, rewards are often helpful. Try keeping a sticker chart. Give your child a sticker for each new thing he tries in a week, and at the end of the week he gets a special prize. You might create a colorful chart of different foods and dishes (use pictures for younger kids) and over the course of a week or a month, have him mark the foods as he tastes them. He wins a reward when he has tasted a certain number of new foods.

Kylee likes to rotate foods (and toys, for that matter). She will eat the same food for a few days and then want to switch, stating she doesn't like it anymore. However, after a week or two "off" the food, she is often excited to eat it again. On the flip side, Jordan says that she doesn't like most foods, but then continues eating them anyway. We haven't quite figured that out, but our point is to keep trying without forcing anything on them.

We also find that by telling Kylee and Jordan what our favorite food is (often in a dramatic way), they both want to imitate us and pretend it is their favorite. So depending on what we would like them to eat, we tell them that it is our "absolute faaaavorite food." They then do the same and ask to eat it as well. The real key here is being dramatic and extreme in our delivery.

When games don't work, creating a scenario where the child has some control can be effective. Let your child pick any dish he wants to have for dinner, as long as it has a new-to-him ingredient in it. Sometimes it's helpful to give him a choice of three suggested dishes, all of which have the target ingredient in them.

It can be frustrating when it seems like no matter what you feed your family, day after day there are strong negative feelings expressed, sometimes loudly, about what you are serving. It is particularly challenging to spend hours preparing a meal only to have your child take a bite, spit it out, and ask for a bowl of cereal instead. Try to stay neutral and take the pressure off him to like everything he eats. Ask him to take a bite, and don't react if he doesn't like it (or spits it out demonstratively). You can sometimes defuse resistance by dealing with it directly: Pin up poster board and list all the dishes or foods you want to try in a month. Keep a running tally of how many family members like a particular item. Maintaining a nameless and blameless atmosphere and keeping it all positive around the topic of dinner can help a reluctant kid feel like part of a community of researchers, rather than a "problem eater."

Please don't infer from what we've said so far that we think you must cook everything from scratch every day. There are many recipes in this book that fit the "quick and easy" profile, and we do urge you to look there for ideas.

But the most important thing is to keep your kid on the healthy food track, so don't worry about using healthy convenience foods, like canned beans, par-boiled whole grains, precooked polenta, and frozen vegetables. Remember that canned beans (ideally without added sodium) are always better than fresh hamburger; try to focus on choosing whole, plant-based foods first, even if it means taking shortcuts.

Last, and perhaps most important, try to keep a sense of humor and per-spective. You won't *always* be negotiating with a 3-, 9-, or 14-year-old!

COVERT OPERATIONS:
IS "HIDING" VEGETABLES NECESSARY?

Of all the different categories of foods in the whole-food, plant-based diet, kids often find vegetables the least appealing to eat, especially when they are served on their own. Thankfully, this book is chockablock with recipes that pair all kinds of vegetables in dozens of different ways with tubers, grains, and beans. A child who considers a side dish of steamed broccoli on her dinner plate an abomina-tion might happily eat that very same broccoli if it's served as part of, say, a tasty stir-fry made with brown rice, black beans, and sauce. Combining veggies with ingredients she loves is a great way to encourage her to eat vegetables. In fact, the veggies often add a nice texture and make a dish more enjoyable.

If your child is particularly resistant to one or more vegetables, just focus on feeding her the ones she *does* like. Don't reject a particular recipe entirely because it has a vegetable in it that your child won't eat. If a recipe for a potato enchilada includes spinach and spinach is a nonstarter for her, replace it with something she prefers. This way your child will enjoy so many more dishes.

For a child who is extremely resistant to vegetables of any kind, try mak-ing them less apparent in dishes by cutting them smaller and adjusting the texture to a different firmness. Another fun way to enjoy different veggies is to serve them as finger foods with her favorite dressing or dip. See page 115 for a recipe that shows how to blanch and shock vegetables such as green beans and broccoli; this preserves their bright color and crunch, and it can make them more palatable to kids than plain raw vegetables.

Remember that it is unnecessary to take the view that your child *must* eat virtually every vegetable, or eat one or more vegetables "from the rainbow" every day. Nor do you have to try to get veggies into every meal or dish. Mashed potatoes and gravy, for instance, do not *need* to be "enriched" with peas or spinach; they provide excellent nutrition all on their own.

That said, if you've tried everything and your child still categorically will not touch most vegetables, it is fine to occasionally "hide" veggies. Cook carrots until they are soft enough to be blended into sauces. Or add greens, cooked and pureed winter squash, grated summer squash, or peas to favorite dishes such as smoothies, muffins, and mac 'n cheese. There is generally little point in doing this for foods your child actually likes. If she happily eats leafy greens, for example, there's no need to make green smoothies solely for the sake of getting yet *more* leafy greens into her. But if your child is having a very hard time getting vegetables from fork to mouth, then go ahead and give a little push in this way.

HAZARD AHEAD: PITFALLS TO WATCH FOR

As we've said, we don't want you to worry about your kid not eating enough. But even if you generally heed that counsel there may still be occasions when shortcuts like excessive ketchup on green beans and vegetable-based processed food can appear to be a very appealing way to get your child to "clean his plate." These are the most common "cheats" we see that can seem great in the short term, but try not to let them become permanent habits.

Liquid calories. The best choice for a drink is water; reserve juice or nondairy milk for a special treat. When we're talking about kids, we don't generally include smoothies in the juice category (nor do we suggest adding juice to the smoothie). Smoothies are blended whole food (unlike juices, which are

OUR STORY:
The (Occasional) Gift of Packaged Foods

The convenience and ease of packaged foods is undeniable (we certainly don't have time to prepare everything from scratch), but in our house we try to limit our own use of them to times of real need. When those moments hit we look for clean packaged foods that can keep Kylee and Jordan entertained long enough for us to get something done, like a load of laundry (otherwise they like to "help" us fold), or enjoy ten minutes of peace to eat dinner. When the girls were babies, we offered them teething biscuits made only from rice and a little sugar and salt. Store-bought pouches of organic fruit-and-vegetable purees were a real boon. Similarly, jars of organic baby food are indispensable. Now that they're older, items made from just a few ingredients, like LÄRABARS, are staples in our pantry. We put this in the category of keeping the larger picture in mind, which is always a good idea when raising children.

extracted) and can be good "kid food" for lean, active children, as well as reluctant eaters. They can also help your child consume lots of healthy fruit. In our house, Kylee fits the profile of someone for whom smoothies are a fine choice. She is lean and active and reluctant to sit down to eat most days, so we prepare smoothies for her when she asks for them (which isn't too often); they're a great way to get a good amount of calories into her and to make sure she's eating some fruits.

While smoothies can be a tasty and nutritious food choice, it is important not to make them a major part of your child's diet. Liquid calories, even in the form of smoothies, are not the most satisfying calories. In making smoothies, the fiber remains present, but it becomes pulverized in the blending process; thus, the smoothie will not fill you up and satisfy your hunger the way unblended whole fruits and vegetables do. This can lead to an inadvertent overconsumption of calories. If excess weight becomes a concern, smoothies, like other liquid calories, should be minimized.

Sweetening food. Sweetening foods to tempt your children to eat can be helpful in the short term to entice a reluctant eater to try new foods, especially when you are transitioning your family to whole-food, plant-based living. But take heed that it may eventually require lots of energy for you to undo the habit. Once a kid gets used to overly sweetened oatmeal, it could take a great deal of time and effort for him to accept oatmeal sweetened only with raisins. Avoid falling into the trap of sweetening almost every food to get your child to eat more because you are worried he isn't eating enough. When you do sweeten foods, we advise using primarily natural sweeteners such as dried fruit, and unsweetened applesauce and other fruit purees and the smallest amount necessary. If you find yourself pouring buckets of maple syrup over rice, you've probably gone too far.

Relying on "kid-friendly" processed meals. As is the case with overly sweetened foods, we can get into trouble when we rely too much on highly processed foods just because we know the kids will eat them. There are a lot of delicious fake meats like "chicken" nuggets on the market. Kids may be drawn to these because of the Dopamine Pleasure Cycle discussed in the Introduction. These hyper-stimulating foods are very appealing to kids and adults alike. And when we serve these foods, our children may indeed eat them, and may consume an arbitrary amount of food we consider "enough." This might seem like a relief when you're dealing with a reluctant eater. But it is not better for a child to eat more of a sweetened or otherwise highly processed food. We'd almost always rather see a child eat less of a whole, plant-based food than more of a processed one. The nutrient value and calorie density of the whole, plant-based food makes it the much better choice.

Avoid ultimatums. When you're introducing a new food, it's best not to tell your child that he cannot have what he really wants until he eats the new item. This is one of the most common ways we see parents unintentionally turning food into a power struggle—one that the parent will almost always lose, incidentally, and at great emotional cost to child and adult alike. What may seem like a reasonable compromise to an adult can seem like the opening salvo in a major ground war to a reluctant child. When you're serving healthy foods, you won't have to battle, because all the choices will be good ones. As discussed earlier, one thing that can be helpful once you've introduced your child to at least a few different foods is to give him a choice among two or three of them. When a child feels he has control over what he eats, he's far less likely to fight about it.

DID YOU KNOW? Calcium alone does not build strong bones. The formula for strong bones depends on two other key factors: getting sufficient vitamin D from exposure to the sun to allow proper absorption of calcium, and regular exercise to build muscle and stress bones in a healthy way.

DO KIDS NEED TO TAKE SUPPLEMENTS?

Vitamins and minerals are vital to proper growth and functioning. Ideally the primary source of them in everyone's diet is plant-based foods. Similarly, the best source for vitamins is food (with the exception of B_{12}, discussed in the next paragraph*). There is no way to know for sure exactly how much of any mineral or vitamin children need on a particular day. Generally it is no more than what a whole-food, plant-based diet will provide. Based on the needs of your child's body, it will absorb more or less of the nutrients supplied by the food she eats. There are some cases when supplementation may be beneficial, but supplements should not be the focus because they are not the basis of good health. We treat supplements like medicine in our practice, as we believe they should be used only in certain circumstances; they should not be taken blindly or abundantly. Instead, the best thing to do is to feed your children whole, plant-based foods.

The exception to this is vitamin B_{12}, the only vitamin we recommend that everyone take, because it is not sufficiently present in non-animal food sources. There is no "perfect" time to begin giving B_{12} supplements to your child, but we usually recommend it when the child starts consuming more solids than breast milk (assuming the breastfeeding mom takes a B_{12} supplement). The best method to administer B_{12} to young children is a lozenge that is easily crushed into a powder so that a small amount of it can be sprinkled on food or offered to her on your finger or in a spoon. We have found that the Jarrow brand works best for our kids and ourselves; it's pretty tasty, so most children accept it happily. We recommend that you talk to your child's pediatrician for specifics on dosage.

---

* Vitamin D is a hormone produced by our body when our skin is exposed to the sun's ultraviolet rays. The best source for vitamin D is to get some sunlight on our skin regularly without burning.

OUR STORY:
A Personal Perspective on Vitamin and Mineral Supplements

Supplementation is often a personal choice that is based on the best scientific evidence available along with how you approach benefit versus risk. We couldn't tell you exactly how much of any one mineral or vitamin our girls get in a day, nor do we know exactly how much either of them even needs on a given day (this actually varies person to person). Instead we focus on the goal of getting them as many of their nutrients as possible from whole plant foods. So over the course of a week we offer our children as many foods as we can from the plant-food groups: fruits, vegetables, tubers, whole grains, and legumes, as well as some nuts and seeds. We also avoid or minimize the harmful stuff such as animal products, added oils, and added sugars or sweeteners. By offering the girls the healthiest food we can and letting them eat when they are hungry, we are confident that in most cases this trumps any supplement we might consider (with the exception of vitamin B_{12}). We also take our girls for regular checkups with a pediatrician we trust. We recommend this approach to our friends, family, and patients, regardless of whether they choose to supplement on top of that, and we recommend you do the same for your children.

FOOD SENSITIVITIES AND ALLERGIES

Given the preponderance of hype that surrounds the issue of food allergies, one could be forgiven for thinking that these are extremely common. In fact, there are relatively few people who have true food allergies and intolerances. A somewhat larger group of people has less potentially dangerous sensitivities to certain foods. The difference may seem inconsequential, but in the medical world it is significant. As doctors, we worry about the fearmongering that sometimes permeates discussions about food sensitivities, making them seem more frightening than the reality warrants. That said, if someone in your family has a true allergy or sensitivity to gluten, the whole-food, plant-based lifestyle is still completely sustainable. Similarly, if a family member is allergic or sensitive to eggs or dairy, you have even more motivation to embrace the whole-food, plant-based lifestyle all the way, a place that is safer not only for the allergic child but also for everyone. Understanding the amplitude of choices and the superiority of these choices in nutrition and health can make it easier to embrace what's possible.

GETTING PERSONAL

Start early, if you can. Explain things to the kids; they are sponges and what they learn, they will carry with them always. Get them involved! Let them help prepare dishes, clean vegetables, and GROW vegetables! Our 8-year-old is into gardening now and has her own. Plus, after eating a more healthy diet, we all feel miserable after eating fast food—and we TALK about it!
—Stacie Merano, Hillsboro, Illinois; three children, ages 8, 16, and 19

Once I find a vegetable that everyone likes, like Swiss chard (thank goodness!), I make sure we have some two to three times a week. I find with the kids, the more they get to "help" in the kitchen with actual food prep—particularly chopping (knives!!! cool!)—the better they eat and the more pride they take in nourishing themselves.
—Cherie Paul, Evergreen, Colorado; two children, ages 9 and 12

To get the boys to eat greens at first I would just hide them in fruit smoothies. After a while they came to like salads, and the younger ones who've been on the diet since birth will eat pretty much any plant-based food I put in front of them.
—Jennifer Beh, Ogden, Utah; five children, ages 3 months, 2, 4, 6, and 8 years

I like to tell my children that eating plants is good for the environment, makes us healthy, and is kind to animals. I try not to say the negative counterstatements, like calling certain foods unhealthy or violent toward animals. Focusing on the reasons not to eat animals would make it harder for my young children when they see their grandparents eating those foods. When I focus on why eating plants is so wonderful, it helps my children understand why we make the food choices we do, without directly addressing the negative consequences of the food choices others around them are making.
—Kelly Caiazzo, Wellesley, Massachusetts; two children, ages 4 and 5

HOW TO HELP YOUR FAMILY MAKE THE FORKS OVER KNIVES TRANSITION

Whether you and your family have been living plant-based for years or are just beginning to consider how to transition, we hope that the previous pages have provided you with inspiration, as well as guidance. If you're completely new to the whole-food, plant-based lifestyle, we offer a few more suggestions in this chapter to help launch you and your family on your journey. Sure, you may meet some hurdles along the way, and this change won't happen overnight. Old habits can be hard to break! But our experience has taught us that once your kids and partner realize that dishes like lasagna, burritos, and mashed potatoes are what's for dinner—and that this lifestyle is most certainly not about eating asparagus all day!—lots of resistance will fall away. At least half the battle is overcoming the false perception that the whole-food, plant-based diet is really hard and is centered on lousy food. The best way to do that is to experience the reality, which is that living this way is all about delicious food shared and eaten together.

If your children are very young, you're likely to have an easier time of transitioning them, since they won't be too attached to unhealthy foods. But if your children are older, from elementary-school age up through high school and beyond, they might need a little more explanation and encouragement, and you might want to be more deliberate about your approach to the transition.

The list of pitfalls to look out for on page 39 can be helpful to you, and here are some specific tips if you're trying to bring along one or more family members who are more set in their ways.

LEARN TOGETHER AND HAVE FUN

Take the burden off yourself to be the sole purveyor of information about whole-food, plant-based living by bringing outside sources in and inviting your whole family to join the discussion. Suggest that you all sit down and watch *Forks Over Knives* or another film together. Buy a book or two, or a few copies of the same book so you can all read at the same time. Our young girls love the Mitch Spinach series of books (see page 274), which are fun to read and informative. Download a podcast and play it on a road trip. There are lots of ways for people at any age to learn more. You want to get the conversation going, and learning together is a good place to begin. See Resources, page 271, for our favorite books, DVDs, and more.

HEAR EACH OTHER OUT

If you want to be successful in implementing any big changes in your family, you need to be attuned to the needs and fears of your children and spouse. Once you get your family involved in the conversation, you have a crucial opportunity to ask them what these are. It may help to review with them the four primary personal needs that come up most often (page xvii).

You may hear needs such as "The food has to taste good," "I don't want to eat strange ingredients," and "I want familiar dishes."

Or, fears such as "I'm worried that my friends will think I'm weird" or "I have so much going on at school/work that I just don't have the bandwidth for changes at home right now."

At the same time, you should freely express your own needs and fears, such as your desire to undertake this change so you feel better, and your concerns about the possibility that your family will make it impossible for you to reach a goal that is important to you. Perhaps it makes sense in your situation to suggest that even if your family doesn't want to do it themselves, they can support something that is important to you (something they're more likely to do if you are clear about your reasons and listen to their concerns).

We find that people sometimes fixate on the strategy, thinking they'll be more successful if they are tactical about implementing the diet. We urge you instead to focus on the connection with the people in your home, and take everyone's needs and fears into consideration. It's about saying to your partner and the others in your house, "Let me try to understand you," and having them do the same. Then ask yourself and each other how you can make it work. (For really recalcitrant family members, see "Don't Let Perfect Be the Enemy of Good," page 54.) It may be best to hold off on moving forward until you are confident that you truly understand all their fears and needs (which may take multiple conversations).

Ideally, no one will dig too deeply into his or her point of view. Remember that it's just as uncompromising for one person to declare that wholesale change is being implemented and there's nothing anyone can do about it as it is for one or more members of the family to adamantly refuse to go along at all. The initiator of the lifestyle stating at the outset, "This is happening because it's better for everyone's health so I won't ever prepare animal products again," is just as upsetting as someone saying, "I will never eat this way so you have to keep making me the same food we've always eaten." The discourse instead should be about connection and compromise, not declarations of what will or will not stand. When you're engaged with your family, nurturing that connection, and open to compromise, you might offer to continue to make a couple of "old" meals a week at the outset, and the rest of the family might agree that they're willing to give it a try. Compromise usually gets people on board more than declarations like "I'm not cooking that for you" or "I'm not eating what you're cooking."

TRY THE GRADUAL APPROACH AND BE FLEXIBLE . . .

Many people successfully implement the lifestyle when they take it slow. Some begin by changing one dinner the first week, then adding another day's dinner each subsequent week. By the end of about two months, they're serving only whole-food, plant-based dinners. Once the dinners are implemented, changing the rest of the meals can happen relatively quickly, since lunches can often be leftovers and breakfasts are generally the easiest to switch over.

Other people decide to begin with a compromise that splits the week evenly. This means three nights whole-food, plant based; three nights omnivore; and one toss-up (often involving leftovers from multiple meals, so that everyone can pick for him- or herself which way to go).

Success with the gradual approach depends on maintaining an open attitude toward the people in your family you're bringing along. Allow them to opt out completely if they really resist what you're serving. (A bowl of cereal or a peanut butter sandwich are some of the best alternatives we know to a fight over food!) If on the whole-food, plant-based nights there is someone who absolutely believes that he can't live without certain animal products, you might say that this is fine, but he'll have to provide these dishes himself. And always suggest delicious alternatives for him to try. A favorite is Almond Dream ice cream for those who love their dish of ice cream after dinner. People are often amazed at how good some alternatives can be. Granted, Almond Dream ice cream is not a health food, but it is a great way to see that dairy isn't the only way to make treats. Once he realizes there are other options that taste good as well, he might be open to trying even healthier ones.

. . . BUT DON'T BE TOO FLEXIBLE

Some parents tell us they want to let their kids try everything, without limitations, so they let them have meat and processed, packaged foods. But these parents surely wouldn't give cigarettes to their kids or offer soda to their toddlers. It doesn't make a lot of sense to give kids choices so that the children

---

DID YOU KNOW? Oil is not a health food. All oil (including olive and every other kind) has more calories per gram than any other food, which means that eating only a very small amount will result in consuming a lot of calories. Oil is 100 percent fat with all other nutrition stripped away, including carbohydrates, protein, vitamins, minerals, fiber, water, and so on. The missing bulk will make it difficult for your body to sense how many calories you have eaten, virtually guaranteeing that you'll eat more calories than you need. Furthermore, all oils have a negative impact on blood vessels and promote heart disease.[12] They may lead to other negative health outcomes, such as suppression of immune system function and increased risk of cancer.[13]

---

don't feel restricted, and then hope the kids will choose the plant foods, because this is not a true choice. It's unfair to the child, given what we know about the Dopamine Pleasure Cycle (see page xv). These foods exploit that system. A kid will almost always pick the higher-calorie-dense, salty, or hyper-sweetened food provided. The pleasure trap is too enticing. Don't set your kid up for a battle she can't possibly win.

ESTABLISH NEW FAMILY HABITS

The family structure depends in part on habits and responsibilities shared by everyone. To reinforce the idea that you can implement new, better habits together, introduce some that you all agree to observe. You can either organize it so that each member of the family comes up with a ritual that the entire family likes or let each family member focus on his or her own. Whatever they are, it is important at first to keep them very simple—like picking a vegetable or two you'll all eat this week—so that they happen no matter what else is going on. After a month or so, when your first very simple habits are established, the family can choose new ones, this time making them a little bit more challenging, like trying oatmeal and fruit for breakfast three out of seven days each week or having cereal with plant-based milk instead of cow's milk a few times a week. As the first few rituals become established, continue this way, gradually making each goal more challenging than the last and trying to make it fulfilling enough that everyone feels a sense of accomplishment when they incorporate it into their lives.

BE PATIENT

As we've said before, it can take many individual introductions of a single food for a child to finally accept it. The more you are exposed to a food, the more likely you are to eat it. This is a good reason to get started! The sooner you begin, the sooner you'll get to where you want to be. But in the meantime, be prepared for your child to merely tolerate new foods rather than wholeheartedly embrace them, at least at first. Don't get discouraged too quickly. Just because he doesn't like black beans during week one doesn't mean he won't like them in a month or two. It's worth trying ingredients in more than one presentation. You can, for example, try presenting black beans in the form of black bean brownies. Some people who won't let a spoonful of lentil soup cross their lips, for instance, find lentil burgers or lentil pasta to be delicious. But if after trying it several times and in different forms your child or partner still just does not like something, don't worry about it. The plant kingdom is vast! Even if your kid never eats Brussels sprouts or lentils in any form, there are plenty of other things to serve for dinner.

FIND A PACE THAT'S COMFORTABLE
FOR YOU AND FOR YOUR FAMILY

It's fantastic if you're so excited about transitioning to the whole-food, plant-based lifestyle that you're ready to get going right away. Just keep in mind that the best pace for a transition depends on the family. Sometimes everyone is on board right away. But sometimes a partner or the kids may not be as gung-ho as you are, and in these cases, a more gradual approach may be better. Your goal is to make changes that last a lifetime, so carefully assess and be mindful of what the personalities in your house can accommodate. But don't let that hinder your personal goals, should you want to move faster for yourself. You're likely to be most successful when you make the transition with foods and meals they recognize. Use their favorite fruits, vegetables, tubers, whole grains, and legumes to make pancakes, burritos, chowder, nacho "cheese" dipping sauce, sloppy joes, and more! And if you need to adapt to individuals' needs during your family's transition phase, try making layered meals such as vegetable lasagna that, once sliced and served, can be sprinkled with cheese by individual diners; a vegetable stir-fry with stir-fried meat on the side that can be added to individual plates; or burritos that you can fill with just beans, or beans and cheese, or meat for those slower-paced family members. And don't forget, if everyone wants to dive right in, just go for it!

NO NEED TO COOK EVERY DAY—
EMBRACE THE REFRIGERATOR AND FREEZER

You might be thinking, "I barely have time to make *one* thing that everyone likes, and now you want me to prepare *multiple* dishes to serve every night?!?"

That is *not* what we are saying. We suggest variety, to be sure, but we don't suggest you prepare all of it at the same time. In our house, most of the food we serve our family is prepared in advance and stored. We spend time on one day off preparing a few dishes in bulk and refrigerate or freeze them. Or we pick a couple of nights a week, when we know we are making a dish that is a family favorite, to make double the amount we'll need for one meal; we eat half and refrigerate or freeze the other half. If you do this in your house, you won't need to cook everything from scratch when it's time for dinner.

FIND A COMMUNITY

A lack of long-term support is one of the biggest reasons people struggle during the transition to, or maintenance of, a whole-food, plant-based lifestyle. Beyond reading books and watching videos at home, we all need community support, and we urge you to look for it in whatever way makes the most sense for you. Thankfully, it gets easier all the time to look out for yourself in this way. Since we began this journey ourselves more than a decade ago, the world has opened dramatically. Today, with just a few clicks of a computer mouse, you can go to sites like Facebook and Meetup.com and find communities dedicated to supporting a plant-based lifestyle. You can meet virtually or face-to-face with people of every stripe, who can exchange recipe ideas, share stories, and even help you through any stumbles. And look at the nonfood communities you're already a part of to find new combinations of people with whom to share your whole-food, plant-based life. Your neighborhood, place of worship, kids' school, and workplace may already have a form of an "eat healthy" campaign—and your whole-food, plant-based lifestyle may fit right in! Also, consider starting your own group-within-a-group (or start a new one from scratch) to share recipes and dishes and to support one another as you blaze new paths in familiar settings.

DON'T LET PERFECT BE THE ENEMY OF GOOD

If you feel like you're getting nowhere with your family, you might be scratching your head and asking yourself a question we professionals often wrestle with: How is it possible that some people still resist implementing the whole-food, plant-based lifestyle even after they understand that it is the single best

---

DID YOU KNOW? We have been led to believe that primarily animal-based foods contain sufficient protein, and that we need to eat those foods to avoid becoming protein deficient. The truth is quite a bit different. Don't worry about not getting *enough* protein; worry about getting too much. Too much protein can lead to kidney stress or damage, kidney stones, calcium loss, osteoporosis, and even, potentially, an earlier death.[14] The amount of protein you need is the amount a diet of whole, plant-based foods provides you. (Mother Nature figured this out well before protein had even been identified!) When you eat a diet based on the main categories that constitute this diet (page xi), you will consume a healthy proportion of protein, which is about 10 percent of your total calorie intake.

---

choice for disease prevention and overall good health? Why won't some people do what they should to get and stay healthy?

Matt's own grandmother once said to him, "Matt, I just can't do your program. I like a steak once in a while." To this common expression of reluctance, we say that we don't care if you have a steak once in a while. The important question is, What do you eat the *rest* of the time?

If you're facing a particularly resistant person in your household, such as an adult or a teenager, perhaps that person, too, has fallen into this all-vegan-or-nothing mind-set. This is not a productive way to think about it. Instead, make some small changes. Our favorite approach with profoundly reluctant people is to ask them to make a very specific "I Won't Change This" list. We ask them to write down everything they will not change. We often see "I won't" statements like:

I won't eat this way during my vacation.
I won't give up cheese on X and Y dishes.
I won't eat collard greens. Or chickpeas.

We encourage them to make as many "I won't" statements as they want, urging them to be as specific as possible. Then we affirm what their list contains so that they know we've heard them. This is an important step with your family members; everyone needs to be heard. After that we declare, "Great, now we can start changing everything else!"

This exercise might seem a little hokey, but it can be successful when other strategies fail. It addresses in a very simple way one of the biggest obstacles to bringing someone along to a new lifestyle: fear of loss of control. Making an "I won't" list lets a person create dispassionate distance between her and something that feels like enormous change. And it allows her to maintain her control over her own choices.

Finally, know that you and your family will probably stumble along the way. Try to see every indiscretion as an opportunity to figure out how someone's needs are not being met, not as an opportunity to harshly judge yourself or the individual. If you've ever tried to meditate, you know that success does not mean that your thoughts never wander. Success is when you get better and better at bringing yourself back to where you want to be after your mind inevitably strays.

GETTING PERSONAL

It was a little rough at first. We were a junk-food, fast-food family. The recipes I used at first were too complicated and foreign. Once I switched to simple whole foods—mashed potatoes, bean burgers and fries, spaghetti, etc.—everything went smoothly.

—Jill Nooe, Grand Blanc, Michigan; two children, ages 13 and 14

Give your children at least a month to turn their taste buds around when offering new foods. My daughter was 3 when I switched from cow's milk to soy and almond. She didn't drink milk for about a month, but eventually made the switch.

—Sandy Ventry, Lincoln, Nebraska; one child, age 19

Every week we have something Mexican, such as burritos, quesadillas, tacos, or enchilada casserole; something Asian, such as stir-fry, kung pao chickpeas, or miso soup; something Italian, like pasta with breaded eggplant, fettuccini cashew Alfredo, or lasagna; a soup, such as lentil, potato leek, broccoli "cheddar," miso, or butternut bisque; a salad, such as kale with crispy tempeh and sesame soy dressing; breakfast for dinner, like waffles, pancakes, or French toast; and a tofu scramble.

—Ali Lipman, Beverly, Massachusetts; two children, ages 6 months and 2 years

I have found enough recipes that work for our family that we have a great variety of dinners. There is always someone who complains about what we're having for dinner, but that was the case before we ate plant-based, too!

—Emily Smith, Red Bluff, California; four children, ages 5, 8, 11, and 15

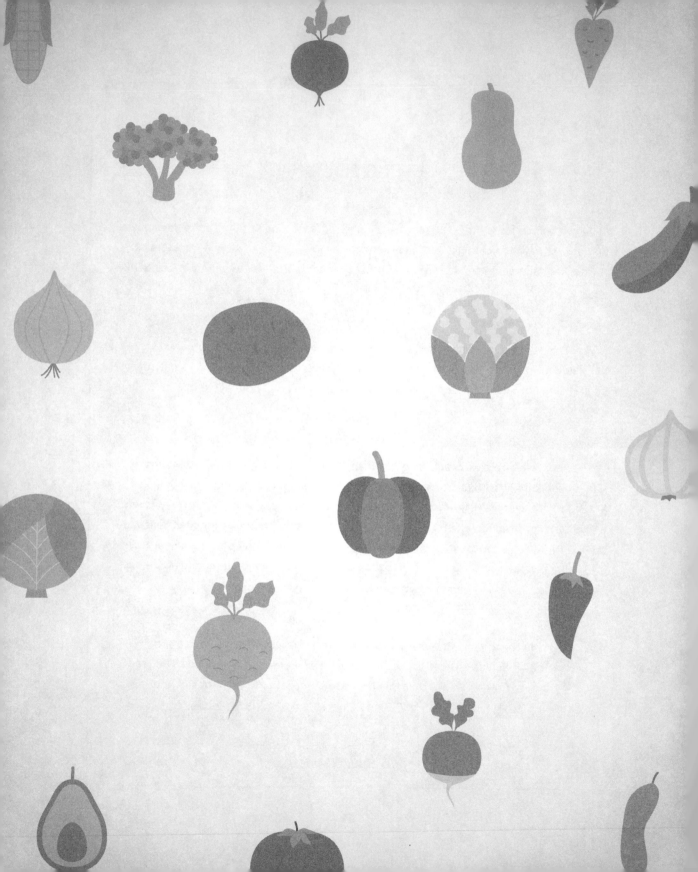

OUT OF THE HOUSE AND ON THE ROAD

For many people living the whole-food, plant-based way, being out of the house can pose challenges that aren't present at home. Whether it's the difficulty of finding an appropriate meal or the inconvenience of dealing with critical outsiders, the world can sometimes feel inhospitable to our lifestyle. But it doesn't have to be that way. Following are some great strategies to make kid parties, Halloween, and even trips to Disney plant-friendly and fun.

Before we dive in, though, we want to stress an important point we made in the last chapter and that we'll reiterate in more detail in the next few pages: don't let perfect be the enemy of good. Our objective is having happy, healthy kids who love to eat and are comfortable in their own skin. This might occasionally mean that we have to hold our tongues when our children make a poor food choice in public. Success is never measured by a single moment in time, and admonishing or otherwise embarrassing your kid about food can really backfire.

SCHOOL LUNCHES

Unless you are one of the very few families in America whose children are enrolled at a school with a sensible understanding of nutrition, we're sorry to say that for the foreseeable future it is unlikely that much, if anything, on the cafeteria lunch menu will be healthy for your kids. That means you'll be packing lunches for many years, so we recommend first that you invest in a good supply of ice packs and check out the lunch-box-friendly recipes in this book. Recipes that are marked this way are generally dishes that store and travel well, so they can be made a day or more in advance and wrapped for packing in a lunch box, or they're dishes that make great leftovers, so the remains of one night's dinner can become the next day's lunch.

If your child is pushing hard to buy a lunch at school that you'd rather she not eat, use what the school will be serving as a jumping-off point to plan lunches to bring. School systems usually give families a monthly meal plan that lists what will be offered for lunch each day. If they'll be serving pizza, chicken wraps, and fish sticks during a week, you can send your child in on various days that week with Quick Mediterranean Pizzas (page 220), a Potato Frankie Roll (page 126), and Red Lentil Fries (page 154) with a dipping sauce or ketchup (all of which you can make for dinner during the week and set aside leftovers for lunches). Again, let your child have input here, so she is making choices. Kids are generally more likely to comply with decisions that they have made themselves.

Sometimes your child can become so determined to buy school lunch that it risks turning into a power struggle. This is very likely an indication she has a need that is not being met. Talk to her to try to figure out what it is; be aware that even *she* might not be sure what her motivations are, so you may have to play detective to help her uncover why she is so eager to do something that clearly goes against her parents' wishes. Is it because she likes the idea of buying her food? Does she want to do what the other kids are doing? Is it that she doesn't want to pack her own lunch anymore? Is the selection of foods generally available for her packed lunch no longer interesting to her? Once you know which of her needs are not being met, you will be better able to address these, which are the underlying cause of her agitation. It may be enough to provide some new lunch options or to offer to help her prepare her lunch for a while. If she's really fixating on buying it, take a look at what's on the menu besides the daily main dish (you may need to contact the cafeteria manager directly). Some schools offer daily à la carte items like hummus, whole-grain crackers, baked fries, salads, and fruit. Offering her the option to buy something that is more within the parameters of your lifestyle might be a compromise that both you and she can live with.

However, if you've tried these approaches and your child still insists that nothing less than buying from the regular menu will work, you might consider letting her do it occasionally. The benefit to this approach, which we recommend you reserve primarily for older children, is that it puts the child in the position of learning for herself. If you go this route, it is important to first discuss with your child, without judgment, what your concerns are, whether it's health, nutrition, morality, or a combination of these. Then let her make her own decision. When she gets home, talk with her about what she ate and how she felt afterwards.

The thing is, there's nothing wrong with letting your kids test their own wings. Frankly, if you insist on making a big deal out of what are essentially minor lapses (an occasional lunch, for instance), your child will only want those "forbidden foods" more. But if you let her make her own choice and use the experience as an opportunity for connecting and learning, you're much more likely to get through to her. In short, whenever possible it's better to let your kids choose themselves not to do something than it is to have them not do something only because you told them that they can't. We've witnessed countless occasions when our kids take a bite or two of something we'd secretly rather they didn't, and then put it down and seek out something far more nutritious, like greens for Kylee or rice for Jordan. Even at one of Jordan's birthday parties, they didn't really eat any of the super-rich foods because those items are not part of their regular diet. And because we don't make any fuss at all about any of these foods, they just aren't that intriguing to the girls. Here's one place where you can really use kids' natural preference for familiar foods to your advantage!

GET INVOLVED TO MAKE THE CHANGE YOU WANT

Having strategies for dealing with the lousy food choices offered at most pre-schools and schools is good, but even better is helping to improve what's of-fered in the first place. The best way to bring about this sort of change is to get involved directly with the PTSA, parent-run boards at private schools, and the administration. We know of "wellness" and "real food" PTSA-affiliated committees at schools that task themselves with lobbying the administration and central offices for better choices at lunchtime, for snacks, and in vending machines. They sometimes also spearhead outreach in the parent community by sharing healthy and tasty recipes on school listservs and supplying lists of great suggestions for parent-supplied treats for birthday and holiday school parties.

So, choose whatever form of involvement works best for you, large or small, because participation of any kind is the surest way to improve the situation for your children. Just remember to keep your communications extremely posi-tive and practical, whether with staff, fellow parents, or kids, and avoid being explicitly critical. You might also reach out to the larger community to invite others to join you. You'd be surprised how willing people are to join a construc-tive and upbeat effort to change the status quo.

KID PARTIES AND OTHER SOCIAL GATHERINGS

Preparation is the best way to ensure that your kids and you can fully enjoy birthday parties and other gatherings you know will involve food. If you're accompanying your child to a party and there is a buffet table, check out that table before your child does, and if necessary ask the host for guidance about which dishes are appropriate. Then you can gently steer your child toward what he can have, rather than allowing him time to focus on what he can't have. This puts you in a position to be able to quickly and positively redirect the ques-tion "Can I have that?" with a concise and direct "We can't have that, but we can certainly have *this.*" In addition, bring an alternative to the birthday cake

OUR STORY:
How Kylee's Preschool Learned the Plant-Based Way

For our part, when Kylee started preschool, we told them that she is allergic to dairy and eggs, and that our family avoided animal products in general for health reasons. We were excited when we got the opportunity to sit down with the director of the center to explain our diet. We gave her a copy of *The Forks Over Knives Plan*, and we asked her to watch the documentary *Forks Over Knives*. She was super-receptive, and she shared the list of snacks served so we could identify what Kylee could and could not eat. Matt spent a couple of hours shopping with staff to suggest alternatives to the items they were already buying, and helped look for ways to buy some products in bulk (so that they can save a little money). In short, we did whatever we could to make it as easy as possible for them to understand the reasons behind why we eat the way we do and learn how to accommodate Kylee, while still ensuring that the entire class had snacks they could enjoy. It helped that they were so open, but they didn't blindly agree. Instead, they tried the food out on the kids and found that they were just as happy with the healthier alternatives. Now they serve foods like rice milk and vegan cream cheese. Some of the snack foods may be a little more refined than we eat at home, but they are shifting in a much healthier direction. Positive encouragement begets positive behavior change. And the best part is the kids really like it and don't miss the less healthy alternatives!

for your child. Make certain that it is something your child really enjoys. It shouldn't feel like a compromise. This is a time to get rich and even a little decadent, so for our girls we usually bring their favorite cookies or chocolate cake. And, of course, there is the option, as we mentioned in our discussion of school lunches (pages 59–61), to simply allow your child to eat the cake that everyone else is eating. It may be the case that a showdown with him at this moment would be more harmful than beneficial in the long term. Instead, you can use it as a learning and connecting experience for you and your child.

If you're comfortable doing so, and especially if you are dropping off an older child at a party you will not be staying for, consider contacting the hosts ahead of time to let them know that you're a plant-based family and offer to bring a treat for your child. In our experience, when this information is presented in a spirit of helpful cooperation, it has always served to relax the hosts by reassuring them that they don't have to go far out of their way to accommodate our children. Furthermore, most hosts are grateful to know in advance what needs their guests (even pint-size ones) have. Once we tell them all of the quick and easy things our kids can eat (such as items on the list on page 32), and they realize how simple it is to support the girls' needs, they usually feel more at ease. Connecting beforehand helps ensure that they'll be able to guide the child toward appropriate foods. And while it isn't possible in every situation, it can be very helpful to offer to bring one of your child's favorite dishes or desserts (in fact, you might want to bring a little extra, because other kids often wind up eating it, too!). This way you know that your child will have something delicious to eat, and even more important, you're creating a smooth path and setting him up for success outside of the house. Plus, you're making it easier for others to accept and appreciate that your dietary choices don't have to be restrictive for them.

For other types of get-togethers for the kids and their friends, such as play dates, it is important to bring or have available richer and more exciting snacks, so that not only your child gets excited to eat them but the other kids want them, too. For our part, we have a bunch of "high-octane" snacks, for occasional

---

DID YOU KNOW? Omega-6 and omega-3 essential fatty acids, which are involved in several important bodily functions and impact blood pressure, inflammation, cancer, and heart disease, should be consumed in a healthy ratio to each other. A diet high in processed and animal-based foods contains an excess of omega-6, which impairs the metabolism of omega-3. The answer is not to eat more omega-3 fatty acids. The answer is to eat a whole-food, plant-based diet, which in most cases restores a healthy omega-6 to omega-3 balance and, more important, leads to positive health outcomes.

---

use, which we keep in a special cupboard above the fridge. These include sweetened cereals that we let the kids have as a dry treat (not for breakfast); rice rolls made with white and brown rice and lightly sweetened; graham crackers; and pretzels. The key here is that these are all foods they already like, which we've made even more special to the girls by designating them as special-occasion-only foods. The enthusiasm for these foods is frankly less about what the foods are than about the fact that we "restrict" the girls' access to them. It's the law of supply and demand: the fact that Kylee and Jordan can have graham crackers only occasionally makes those graham crackers precious commodities. These valuable kid treats also include homemade cookies and juice Popsicles that we offer when Kylee has a friend over to play. She gets very excited when we pull any of these out on our way to or during a play date. All of this goes a long way toward normalizing the plant-based diet for your kids and the people who surround them, which is naturally our long-term goal.

HALLOWEEN AND OTHER CANDY-CENTRIC EVENTS

The culinary traditions of most major holidays can be easily tweaked to accommodate the plant-based lifestyle (the answer is almost always to bring a big

OUR STORY:
Hosting Plant-Based, Kid-Friendly Parties

When we host birthday parties at our house, we never have an issue putting together a spread of food that can please kids and parents alike while staying completely within our parameters. Pretty much everyone can find something he or she will enjoy on a table that holds things like a big platter of cut-up fruit; a tray with veggies and Ranch Dressing (page 242); hummus and bean dip served with chips or crackers; and big bowls of Herbed Popcorn (page 106). As for the mandatory cake, we have a favorite vegan bakery near us that creates wholly plant-based, oil-free delectable ones. Increasingly though, living near something so specialized is not necessary. More and more mainstream bakeries will easily (and deliciously!) accommodate all sorts of dietary restrictions and allergies. Many can work completely within your guidelines, and others can get pretty close, which is fine for a once-in-a-while event. Or if you prefer to prepare something yourself, take a look at the selection of celebration-worthy desserts in this book, all of which are consistent with the whole-food, plant-based lifestyle.

Hosting events away from home—for instance, at popular kid party spots like bowling alleys, laser tag and paintball venues, trampoline parks, moon-bounce centers, and sports complexes—can be more challenging. This is because many of these places require that they provide all the food served, which invariably means a selection of some of the worst Standard American Diet fare there is. We counsel you to bypass those "standard" offerings and speak directly to someone at the site, ideally a manager. We've found it easiest in these contexts to describe our restrictions simply as allergies. (Don't worry about trying to persuade them of the advantages of the diet. Instead, focus on collaborating with the staff on a menu you can be comfortable eating and serving to your kids.) We always begin by asking if we can bring our own food. If this isn't possible, and it often isn't, we suggest the ways they can accommodate us within *their* parameters—for example, cheese-free pizza; chips and salsa; and dairy-free ice cream. We've found that the kids enjoy these kinds of choices enormously during the 3½ minutes they're not engaged in whatever activity the site specializes in, which is the point of having a party off-site in the first place!

dish or two to share). But there are a few candy-centric holidays such as Halloween and Valentine's Day that loom so large in the kid universe that it can be hard for parents to help their children resist the inexorable pull of mountains of junk food. This is especially true when aisles of brightly wrapped treats appear in stores more than a month before the actual holidays! There are a few different ways to ensure that your kids enjoy all the fun that comes with these special days without forcing you to completely abandon your principles. And these approaches can be used to deal with other candy-loaded events, such as the piles of piñata-booty plus goody-bag loot that come home after many birthday parties.

The first thing to do is to allow your children to participate in the holiday *activities*, such as trading valentines and going trick-or-treating. The part that you want to focus on is the candy and junk that follows the active portion of these days. You can take the path of least resistance and make it a one-time-only affair, where your children can have what they want on the day or night of the holiday, and then the rest goes away. This is not our first choice, but many parents, especially those who are transitioning with older children, find this to be the best, most workable solution for events that come up just a few times in a year. For our part, we like the "Switch Witch," especially on Halloween. Our kids go trick-or-treating with the rest of the neighborhood and their friends. That night they bundle up all their candy and leave it out for her when they go to bed. When they wake up the next morning, they'll find that the "Switch Witch" has taken their candy and left a present in return. We also have used candy as currency to buy toys and treats, which can be fun. For example, a small "Shopkins" toy can cost three mini candy bars while a new doll costs twenty pieces of regular candy; you can make this even more elaborate based on the age and interests of your child.

Whether one of these or another tactic works best for you naturally depends on the people in your family and your personal circumstances. No matter which approach you take, if you and your children do observe these holidays, we urge you to focus on creating an atmosphere that allows your kids to feel

---

DID YOU KNOW? Sugar as it occurs in whole foods supports human health. It's a problem only when it is extracted from its natural package and used to excess. The extraction, or refining, process removes the water, fiber, and virtually every other nutrient of the food. In this state it is more calorie dense and thus overstimulating to our pleasure senses (see page xv). (Note that small amounts of added sugar, especially in food made at home, can be enjoyed occasionally without posing significant health risks.)

---

free to participate in the camaraderie and festivity of these special days. Present your adaptations as part of the celebration and your children will see them that way, too.

AMUSEMENT PARKS AND OTHER EXTRAVAGANZAS

If you've read everything we've written up to this point, you won't be surprised to hear us say that advance preparation is the best road to success when traveling—be it for a day or a week—to an amusement park or other family-friendly venue. When the most plentiful "kid foods" advertised at these places are chicken nuggets and pizza, it does require a little extra time and effort to ensure that your family can fully participate in the fun without compromising your principles—or going home with very upset stomachs.

When traveling someplace where we'll be staying overnight, our first priority is finding a place to stay that has a kitchen (many family-friendly hotels offer this accommodation). Then we shop at a local grocery store and cook some of our meals in the hotel, which not only helps us stay healthy but also saves us a lot of money. We bring some auxiliary food from the grocery store with us to the park, and most places offer fruit, salads, or smoothies for snacks.

When we've gone to places like Disney World, for the meals we eat out we try to call the restaurant ahead of time to make sure they can have available plain baked potatoes and salads with no cheese or dressings. Then we bring our own condiments, like ketchup, honey mustard, guacamole, and hummus. This way we can sit at the restaurant like everyone else, but we are still eating within our guidelines. Calling ahead can make it easier for you at big, busy places with lots of stimuli, where your kids are more likely to start begging for foods you definitely don't want them to eat before you can figure out what's on the menu. But if you don't call ahead, it's usually pretty easy to look at a menu and figure out your options. Here, as elsewhere, we advise against looking at a menu and telling your kids what they can't have. Instead, tell them what they *can* have. Most restaurants (even the fast-food counters that are so common at big "family-friendly" venues) have one or more items like pasta, steamed grains, baked potatoes, and steamed or raw vegetables. It is also easy to get breads and/or corn tortillas when out in many restaurants, along with hummus, guacamole, vinegars, salsas, soy and sweet sauces, ketchup, and mustards to add some flavor to the side dishes. Another trick is to use soup (confirm it is made with vegetable stock) as a sauce. Don't hesitate to point out to the wait-staff what they have listed on the menu as sides or accompaniments to other dishes and ask them to simply serve you a combination of those. A couple of our favorite tricks in restaurants are to pour bean or vegetable soup over a baked potato or stir steamed rice into the soup. The goal here, of course, is to eat, but also to teach your kids how to advocate for themselves and to allow them to feel part of the action at a fun restaurant without undermining your values.

Finally, as we touched on earlier and will elaborate on a little more in the next section, don't worry about being perfect. It can be hard on anyone, and especially parents, to make sure that in every single situation you're eating absolutely pure, oil-free food. Sometimes when you're on the road, your options are limited—yet you still need to eat! In our family, we always avoid animal foods. But we frankly don't fret over occasional white rice, white pasta, or even oils, especially when we're traveling.

OUR STORY:
The Forks Over Knives–Friendly Disney Character Breakfast

When we took the girls to Disneyland one summer, setting up a character breakfast required only a little extra planning, but it was well worth it. We asked the booking agent in advance if they could accommodate dietary restrictions and confirmed that we'd like to discuss them with the chef when we arrived. They were extremely accommodating, and when we arrived the chef came out so we could explain our restrictions. He came up with many options, including vegan Mickey Mouse waffles, special home fries without oil, and vegan sausages that were not processed. In addition, he pointed out all the options already on the menu that we could eat, and he sent out big bowls of fresh fruit for our oatmeal instead of the small amount of fruit cocktail on the buffet table. We wound up looking like gluttons! Other diners might even have been a little jealous at the sight of our table laden with bowls of bright, fresh food. Needless to say, Kylee and Jordan were very happy and able to fully enjoy this experience. And what made it extra special for us was seeing the girls try all these foods, and then go back to what was familiar (and ultimately healthiest). For Kylee it was oatmeal and fruit, while Jordan enjoyed her steamed rice and avocado enormously—just like at home! We never stop being delighted when we see Kylee and Jordan being naturally drawn to their good-for-them staple foods.

FOCUS ON THE BIG PICTURE

Our goal is for your child to adopt a healthy diet for a lifetime. This means, somewhat contradictorily, that we occasionally have to overlook digressions. In other words, we want to keep our focus on the 90 percent, not the 10 percent. To do this we lay the groundwork by teaching our kids why we eat the way we do: for health reasons, to help protect animals and the environment, and because we feel good when we eat this way. Kids who are armed with straightforward information and who receive honest answers from us are most likely to ultimately decide on their own to embrace whole, plant-based foods. Your job is to educate, support, and do your best.

Denying your child cake at a friend's birthday party may seem like a win in the short term, but it can breed resentment and lead to rebellion and ultimately all-out failure. In a situation in which your child is absolutely determined to eat the same cake that everyone else is eating, we recommend not digging in. Instead, remind her to be careful not to eat too much or too quickly, or she might get a stomachache, and gently remind her to pay attention to how she feels after eating the cake. We often see in these situations—which can quickly become more about control than food choices—that children simply want a bite of the cake, not to finish the whole thing (especially when well fed prior to the party; try to be sure your child goes to all events well fed so she isn't ravenous from the start). As long as the food in question is not seriously harmful (because the child has a true allergy, for instance), the key is to inform and then support her, even if you don't approve of the decision. When you feel the time is right at some point after the event, you might talk about it with your child and help her process whether the pros of her choice outweighed the cons. Help her imagine what other choice she could have made in that moment. Was there fresh fruit available, for instance, or would she like it if there could be an alternative that she brings with her to future birthdays; or, if you brought an alternative that she rejected, how could that situation be fixed?

And when your teenager wants to go to a fast-food restaurant because "all her friends" are going, remind her that even at McDonald's you can get food that is at least vegan; and then try not to fret if she eats the nonvegan options her friends eat. The bottom line with teenagers is that you cannot force them to eat exactly what you want them to in every situation. Helping our children learn to make good choices for themselves is more effective, we believe, than forcing our choices onto them. There is an enormous benefit to focusing more on explaining why your family eats the way you do than on demanding that your child observe every boundary in every setting.

"YOU FEED YOUR KIDS *WHAT?*": HOW TO HANDLE CRITICISM FROM OTHERS

When faced with skepticism about the educated diet and lifestyle choices we have made for ourselves, it might be easy to find the words and positive attitude to push back. But when someone makes us feel defensive about our choices for our children, it can be much more difficult to respond proportionally. And it's especially painful when the skeptic is someone we trust, such as a caring family member or our child's pediatrician.

If you find yourself in this position, remember (and point out, if you'd like) that it makes no sense that a diet you know is good for adults would be unhealthy for kids. The fact is that in generation after generation, most kids eat the way their adult caretakers do. Today, after decades of the Standard American Diet, the result is an epidemic of childhood obesity. It can seem illogical that you should have to justify your diet over the diet that is obviously making people very sick. Yet we've all found ourselves in this situation. Short of shaking your head and walking away, here are a few dependable approaches to handling these kinds of encounters.

You may be surprised to hear that in certain cases the best first line of defense is no defense at all. Simply letting a challenge to your lifestyle choices pass you by without responding directly will get you further than you think. If nicely deflecting a question is unrealistic or uncomfortable, at the very least do your best not to internalize the questioner's implied or explicit criticism.

Sometimes knowing what *not to say* is more important than knowing what *to say*. When you feel compelled to engage, you can reassure your questioner that there's a wealth of evidence about the vast benefits of the whole-food, plant-based lifestyle; you've researched the subject; and most compelling of all, you've seen the benefits in your own life and are confident in your point of view. Sometimes caring family and friends just need a little reassurance; remember that your parents love your kids, too. Assure them that you'd never jump into this without doing your homework. (And you can rest assured that we've done our homework, and we know for sure that plants are best for kids!).

Sometimes it helps to respond to direct questions with questions of your own; this can help create a balance in the discourse. You might ask them for evidence to support their recommendations and then offer the evidence you have for a whole-food, plant-based diet. If their concerns are that they don't think there is evidence to support your choices, then you can easily suggest any of the multiple sources of information listed on page 271. Information about and support for whole-food, plant-based living come in all kinds of media— books, pamphlets, websites, DVDs, YouTube videos, podcasts, and smartphone apps. There truly is something for everyone!

Some people may express concerns that the action of growing teeth, bones, and brains requires substantively different nutrients and thus a different diet from what adults need. While it is true that the body needs different amounts of nutrients at different times of life, it is equally true that the whole-food, plant-based diet is most consistent with everyone's needs, whether child or adult.

We find that the root of most challengers' objections is a preconceived notion they have of what terms like "vegan" or "whole-food, plant-based" mean, and that the perceived "otherness" of these ideas equates to insufficiency. If you break down for them what you and your kids eat, rather than allowing a continued focus on what they *don't* eat, they may be able to better understand. So, you can say that your kids eat fruit (yes, that is healthy); vegetables (oh yes, that is healthy, too); beans and legumes (yup, still healthy); whole grains (healthy); and some nuts and seeds (wow, still healthy). Better still, point out some of the familiar dishes you all enjoy. Most people we know can appreciate pizza, mashed potatoes, burritos, pasta and red sauce, and pancakes!

If your questioner is someone with whom you'd truly like to connect over this issue—perhaps it's a family member or a close friend you see a lot and who might resist because he sees your lifestyle choice through the prism of how it will affect his life—you might want to offer to sit down at another time and show him your own trusted sources for information about the whole-food, plant-based lifestyle. We suggest moving the conversation to a different time and place because, in our experience, we get very little accomplished when we're put in a position of defending something on the spot and when there are other people around. You're often better able to have a productive conversation in another venue. By the way, moving the conversation to another place and time is a good idea even when you're ready and eager to tout the benefits of the whole-food, plant-based lifestyle on the spot. It's important to gauge your audience to determine if he is ready and willing to be open to whatever you want to share. If you do offer information, be mindful of your surroundings and listener, and keep your delivery upbeat and nonjudgmental. Remember that in certain settings, your enthusiasm—which we share—can seem as off-putting to people as their skepticism can seem to you. If you're feeling really great and your kids are healthy and thriving, that is evidence enough to demonstrate to others the wisdom of your lifestyle.

GETTING PERSONAL

We try to create a fun, happy environment around food, not anything that is about sacrifice but about abundance. We celebrate holidays with many traditional foods, but we just make them vegan. It is especially challenging for young people who are still developing their voices to be challenged by a group of teasing peers. Subvert that by creating your own community that supports how you live and eat.

—Marla Rose, Berwyn, Illinois; one child, age 13

For my children it's our "normal," but the biggest challenges come from the judgment of others—that we are somehow denying our children the basic human right to a McDonald's burger. It is difficult for the kids not to be affected by that when it comes from their friends, but now that they are of an age to be reasoned with, they watch DVDs (such as *Forks Over Knives*) that help to confirm to them that they eat the best way possible. Of course, that positive dialogue is ongoing.

—Karen Neave, North Island, New Zealand; two children, ages 11 and 13

PART II

THE FORKS OVER KNIVES FAMILY RECIPES

As parents, we have been happily raising a Forks Over Knives family for several years, and as doctors we've been eagerly advocating the lifestyle for even longer. One thing we know for sure after all this time is that the best way to make it work is to have a great selection of easy and delicious recipes. For those, we turn to our good friend and resident Forks Over Knives Culinary Projects Manager, Darshana Thacker. We're delighted to turn over the pen to her here so that she can share with you her invaluable tips for building and maintaining an efficient whole-food, plant-based kitchen and more than 125 excellent, kid-friendly recipes.

FORKS OVER KNIVES FAMILY RECIPES
BY DARSHANA THACKER

I've loved to be around food since I was a child. Some of my favorite memories are of watching and helping the women in my family prepare one delicious vegetarian dish after another during our summer holidays in my mother's hometown near Mumbai, India. After I immigrated to the United States in 2001 I transitioned to a fully plant-based diet, adapting the skills and recipes I learned at the elbows of those wise women to my oil-free, plant-based kitchen.

I also studied at the Natural Gourmet Institute in New York City, one of the top professional vegetarian culinary schools in the country, where I learned modern and traditional cooking techniques from around the world. The food I make from whole, plant-based ingredients incorporates the range of cuisines I was exposed to in my childhood, through my travels, and at school. My goal is to show how easy it is to prepare great-tasting, plant-based meals and to help make living this way accessible to more and more people every day.

I am thrilled to have put all of my training and experience to work to develop the recipes that follow, and I did so with kids just like yours in mind. These recipes use common ingredients to appeal to kids' less-adventurous palates and are generally quite simple to prepare, yet they are varied enough in taste and texture to please adults. But before we dive in and start cooking, I hope you'll take a few minutes to read this brief introduction to my favorite ingredients, kitchen tools, and techniques. Included are some great tricks for maintaining an efficient kitchen—one where you'll be happy to cook, because you have what you need to make easy and stress-free meals.

PANTRY, FRIDGE, AND FREEZER STAPLES

These are the ingredients that are staples of a plant-based kitchen.

Plant milk

It's surprisingly simple to make your own almond milk (page 264) and buy soy milk made only from soybeans and water (Westsoy and Edensoy both make good versions), but this is not always feasible in every kitchen. When buying store-bought plant milk, look for brands with as few ingredients as possible, and the best choice is unsweetened and unflavored. Many store-bought plant milks have vanilla flavoring in them, which is generally fine if you're using the milk in a dessert, but the flavoring will ruin most savory dishes. No matter how adventurous your taste buds may be, vanilla and pesto just don't go well together.

Sweeteners

For a great all-around general-use sweetener, a good choice is date paste. It is very easy to make (page 265) from just dates and water, and it can be stored in the refrigerator or freezer for several months. It can be used both in savory cooking and baking, and it adds a nice but not cloying sweetness. Applesauce, bananas, and other fresh fruit purees are also wonderful natural sweeteners. When more concentrated sweetening is desired, small amounts of pure maple syrup do the trick nicely.

Spices and Dried Herbs

A thoughtfully stocked spice cabinet will help ensure that even the simplest dish you prepare has outstanding flavor.

- Ground allspice

- Basil

- Bay leaves

- Black pepper

- Cayenne

- Chile powders: *Rather than using a generic "chili powder," take advantage of how many wonderful dried chiles are now widely sold ground. Some good ones are ground ancho, pasilla, New Mexico, and arbol powder. Pick a couple that you like and keep them handy, especially for Mexican dishes.*

- Ground cinnamon

- Ground cloves

- Ground coriander

- Ground cumin and cumin seeds

- Ground fennel seed

- Garlic powder

- Lemon peel: *Adds zesty lemon flavor and is great to have on hand when you need citrus flavor but you're out of fresh lemons.*

- Marjoram

- Nutmeg

- Onion powder

- Oregano

- Parsley

- Rosemary

- Sage

- Salt: *We suggest that you use minimal salt in general. In most recipes it's added at the end of cooking so that the dish does not become overly salty. Sea salt and pink salt are preferable to ordinary table salt.*

- Smoked paprika: *Great for adding a bit of smoked flavor to a dish.*

- Sweet or mild paprika

- Tarragon

- Thyme

- Ground turmeric

- White pepper: *Made from the same berries as black pepper but with the outer layer removed. White pepper is hotter and more pungent than black.*

Spice blends

A blend of several herbs or spices can add layers of flavor to a dish. Some wonderful spice blends are curry powder, Italian seasoning, herbes de Provence, and Mild Creole Seasoning (page 169). Having these spice blends on hand makes it very easy to create a new, flavorful meal using leftover produce, pasta, grains, or cooked beans.

Flours

Having a few different flours in the freezer (the best place to store them) allows you to create a rich variation of texture and flavor in your baked goods. You don't need to have all the flours in the following list to make the recipes in this book; as long as you have all-purpose and whole wheat flours, you can make almost anything here. But adding at least one or two different flours to your own collection will open up new and interesting flavor and texture possibilities. And for people keeping a gluten-free kitchen, gluten-free grain flours are essential. Note, though, that even if the product you are buying is naturally gluten-free (as corn is, for example) look for products specifically labeled "gluten-free" to avoid cross-contamination.

- **All-purpose**: Neutral. Not gluten-free. Use in place of any flour listed here. Can itself be replaced with buckwheat, or oat, sorghum, or quinoa flour, and in part by whole wheat flour.

- **Almond and cashew**: Nut flavor. Gluten-free. Almond and cashew flours are excellent sources of whatever fat is required in baked goods. Products labeled "meal" are generally coarser than those that are labeled "flour," although sometimes the labels are used interchangeably.

- **Barley**: Neutral flavor. Not gluten-free; however, barley flour has only a small amount of gluten, so it can't be used in place of wheat flour if making leavened bread and it is always used in combination with other flours in baked goods.

- **Brown rice flour**: Slight nutty taste. Gluten-free. Because brown rice flour is gelatinous when cooked, it's good to use in desserts such as puddings.

- **Buckwheat**: Strong nutty flavor. Gluten-free. Works well as a wheat substitute in baking and for making pancakes.

- **Chickpea**: Nutty flavor. Gluten-free. Chickpea flour has a distinct flavor that makes it great to use in cooking. When used in baking, it's better to combine it with another, neutral flour.

- **Corn flour, cornmeal, polenta**: All have distinct corn flavor. Gluten-free. Corn flour is a refined product used in small quantities to bind (hold together) batters and doughs. Cornmeal is whole grain and comes in a variety of grinds from fine to coarse. It is also a good, whole-grain replacement for bread crumbs. Polenta is coarse-ground cornmeal.

- **Oat**: Light flavor. Gluten-free. Oat flour is used as a thickener and as a substitute for whole wheat flour in combination with other flours, such as sorghum, quinoa, and cornmeal.

- **Quinoa**: Neutral flavor. Gluten-free. Quinoa can be used in combination with oat flour or buckwheat to replace whole wheat flour to make gluten-free baked goods.

- **Rye**: Deep, distinct flavor. Not gluten-free. Whole-grain dark rye flour can replace whole wheat flour for a denser texture and rich flavor. Balanced with all-purpose flour, it can give you a lighter texture than whole wheat flour will.

- **Sorghum**: Very neutral flavor, light texture. Gluten-free.

- **Spelt**: Light flavor. Not gluten-free. Spelt, a kind of wheat, makes a flour with a milder flavor than whole wheat.

- **Whole wheat**: Deep wheat flavor, dense texture. Not gluten-free. Whole wheat flour can replace a portion of many flours, but it's heavier than most so don't overdo it. For best results, don't replace more than one-fourth of the total amount of all-purpose or other flour with whole wheat flour.

USEFUL TECHNIQUES FOR OIL- AND DAIRY-FREE COOKING

Cooking without oil, eggs, or dairy has so many advantages, not least of which is how much faster it is to clean up when you're finished! A few simple techniques make it easy to do things like sauté vegetables and create creamy sauces without oil or cream.

Cooking vegetables

To cook large vegetables such as sweet potatoes or beets, roasting or steaming are good options (see page 89). For dishes that involve sautéing ingredients like onions, garlic, or peppers, water or vegetable stock serve the role that oil does in conventional cooking. Begin cooking chopped vegetables with a bit of liquid. Keep an eye on them as they cook and add liquid 1 to 2 tablespoons at a time. This creates just enough steam to keep the vegetables from sticking, yet prevents the dish from getting too wet. This is less necessary with vegetables that are very moist, so you won't see this reminder in every recipe.

Often, vegetables are cooked on their own before being added to a dish. It is generally unnecessary to bring large pots of water to a boil to quickly cook a small amount of vegetables. Instead, you'll see on these pages that veggies are often boiled in a relatively small amount of water. It cuts back on water use and saves a little time, plus the concentrated cooking liquid is often flavorful after the veggies are drained. This remaining cooking liquid can be used to cook grains or beans, can serve as the base for soups and stews, or, as just described, can be added to prevent sautéing vegetables from sticking to the pan.

Flavor enhancers

For bright flavor in salad dressings, try citrus or fruit juice, vinegars, low-sodium tamari or soy sauce, and small amounts of nut butters. For deeper flavor, use vegetable stock instead of water when cooking grains, soups, stews, and sauces.

Almonds or cashews add creaminess to soups and sauces, replacing the need for cream. Soak the nuts in water to soften them and then blend them with the liquid until smooth. Stir this paste into soups or sauces to add a lovely creamy texture.

Baking and desserts

To bind batters and doughs, and achieve a nice crust on baked goods, use plant milk, date paste (page 265), fruit juice, fruit pulp, and small amounts of nut butters and nut flours.

TIPS FOR MAINTAINING AN EFFICIENT KITCHEN

By spending just a little bit of time once in a while preparing a few basic and often-used ingredients, you will save yourself much more time and energy on busy evenings.

Garlic and ginger

The aroma and flavor of garlic and ginger bring life to many dishes, but it can be tedious to mince them every time they are called for in a recipe. This is the kind of chore that can easily dissuade tired people from cooking on a busy weeknight. Instead, invest a little time mincing a large quantity of these ingredients and freezing them in ice trays. Once frozen, you can transfer the cubes to airtight containers and keep them in the freezer for up to one month.

Whenever a recipe calls for minced garlic or ginger, all you have to do is reach in and pull out a cube or cut part of a cube off—it'll defrost in just a few minutes (although you don't have to wait for it to do so to use it). The recipes in this book include volume equivalencies for every ingredient, so you can easily pull out just the amount you need. For your reference, one clove of garlic is equivalent to ½ teaspoon minced and a 1-inch piece of ginger will give you 1 teaspoon grated. (Note that it's not necessary to peel ginger before using, but if you prefer to, it's absolutely fine to do so.)

Grains, beans, and legumes

Whole grains, beans, and legumes are such an important part of the plant-based diet that it's likely you'll eat some or all of them daily. This doesn't have to mean, though, that you must cook them daily. Instead, you can prepare a big batch of one or two grains and one or two beans or legumes, and store them in the fridge or freezer so they are ready for meals all week long (they'll keep for four to five days in the refrigerator or up to one month in the freezer). One key for making this system very usable is to divide the batch into smaller portions and store them in glass containers. For instance, many recipes call for 15-ounce cans of beans, which is the equivalent of 1½ cups cooked beans. Divide the batch of beans into 1½ - or 3-cup portions before freezing so that you can easily remove just the right amount as you need it.

To thaw grains, place the glass container without the lid in a steamer for 15 to 20 minutes. They get soft and fluffy. To thaw beans, run hot water over the glass container with the lid in place; to thaw them more quickly, you may run the hot water directly over the beans.

A note on rinsing beans and grains: It can be easy to forget when we buy whole beans and grains in sealed containers that they are a natural food, just like fresh produce, and should be well rinsed before cooking. The best way to rinse beans is to put them in a strainer and run cold water over them, raking through them with your fingers and discarding shriveled or discolored ones. To rinse grains place them in a large bowl and cover with a generous amount of water. Swish them around several times, then drain in a mesh strainer. Repeat a few times until the water is clear. Drain thoroughly before cooking.

Fresh herbs

Keep one or two bunches of cleaned fresh herbs like cilantro and parsley in the fridge to use as a garnish and to freshen up leftovers and reheated frozen dishes. Wash the whole bunch and dry thoroughly in a salad spinner or spread on a baking sheet or tray lined with a kitchen towel and let stand 15 to 20 minutes until dry. Wrap the herbs in paper towels and store in a plastic container with a tight-fitting lid; the washed sprigs will last four to five days. This makes it much easier to pull out a few sprigs to chop and add to a dish. You can also chop a small amount in advance and store in an airtight container in the refrigerator, but once chopped, fresh herbs will last only about one day.

Citrus juice

Fresh lemon and lime juices contribute bright flavor to so many plant-based dishes and dressings that it's a very helpful time-saver to have jars of juice at the ready. Every couple of weeks you can juice about ½ cup of each (from roughly 8 lemons and 8 to 10 limes) and store in mason jars in the refrigerator. The juices will keep for two to three weeks.

INVALUABLE TOOLS FOR OIL-FREE COOKING

No special equipment is necessary for oil-free cooking, but a few inexpensive kitchen tools will certainly make life a little easier.

Heat or flame diffuser

Oil-free cooking means that we can't rely on added fats to keep cooking foods from sticking to the bottom of the pan. Adding a little water or vegetable stock works well in many cases, but sometimes these additions can throw off the balance of the dish. A heat diffuser, which distributes the heat evenly across the entire pan and keeps it low and gentle, is an effective tool for keeping food from sticking.

Blender

A very useful part of a well-stocked plant-based kitchen, a blender makes smooth, oil-free sauces, soups, and marinades. Plus, almost every fruit can be frozen and transformed into delicious ice "cream" in minutes. All the recipes in this book were developed using a standard $20 blender, so you don't need a blender with an extra-powerful motor to prepare these dishes. If you are using a more powerful blender, the recipes will certainly work; you may need a little less liquid and/or time to reach the desired result.

Nonstick skillet or griddle

Most dishes can be prepared in almost any pot or pan no matter what the finish is. However, for dishes such as pancakes, a good-quality nonstick skillet or griddle is crucial.

Large steamer or steamer basket

Steaming is often the best way to cook large vegetables such as potatoes and beets, and a specific tool for this task makes it easier. A dedicated steamer pot is helpful but not necessary. An inexpensive expandable steamer basket is just as good, and it can fit into almost any pot, from a wide sauté pan to a taller saucepan.

Silicone baking mats and cupcake molds

Probably the single biggest challenge in oil-free cooking is preventing baked goods from sticking to the pans they are cooked in. Flat silicone mats for lining baking sheets and silicone cupcake molds practically eliminate this problem. They are flexible, durable, and in my experience, almost nothing sticks to them.

Parchment paper

Parchment paper is great for transforming regular baking surfaces (baking sheets, cake pans) into nonstick surfaces quickly and inexpensively. Rolls of parchment are available at any grocery store, but if you have the room, buy a box of parchment precut to the size of your baking sheets. This is enormously convenient. You'll find the best prices for this (and other baking supplies) at a dedicated baking or restaurant supply store.

Pressure cooker and rice cooker

These two specialty items are not called for in the recipes that follow, but they are useful tools to have in a plant-based kitchen. The pressure cooker cuts down the time it takes to cook dried beans, soups, and stews, and rice cookers turn cooking whole grains into a "set it and forget it" task—a real boon in busy households.

A FEW NOTES ON THE RECIPES

Most recipes yield a large portion, both because they are designed for families and because they are good as leftovers or for freezing for future meals.

- One of the best parts of cooking dinners at home is using leftovers for lunch the next day, but not every dish lends itself to refrigerator storage and lunch-box packing. There are plenty of dishes in this book that do, however, and they are marked with a ⬢ . Store these as indicated at the end of the recipe, and enjoy that home-cooked goodness even when you're away from home!

- A big key to starting and maintaining a whole-food, plant-based, oil-free kitchen is building a well-stocked pantry, refrigerator, and—almost the most important thing of all—freezer. When you have already prepared sauces, soups, beans, or grains in storage, meal prep can be done in a fraction of the time. Storage times are listed at the end of every recipe that can be stored for days or even months either in the refrigerator or freezer. This is helpful information for dealing with leftovers, to be sure, but even more than that, it's an invaluable resource for stocking your freezer. Whenever you cook something that's a good "storer," make a double batch and freeze half. You'll thank yourself later!

- Another great aspect of having extra food prepared is that from just a few parts (cooked potatoes, frozen vegetables, and a delicious sauce, for instance) you can pull together a meal very quickly. The "Quick and Easy" chapter holds some of our favorite ways to use leftovers and my freezer staples. Make the recipes just as written, or use them as jumping-off points and inspiration to create your own new creations using up whatever leftovers are in *your* fridge.

Now let's get cooking!

RECIPES

BREAKFAST

Chocolate Chip Coconut Pancakes 📷

Makes about 8 (4-inch) pancakes ■ *Ready in 25 to 30 minutes*

These pancakes are so simple and delicious, and they're just as good for dessert as they are for breakfast! Plus, they freeze really well, so you can make an extra batch and freeze them. Use a large griddle so that you can cook three or four at a time.

1 tablespoon flaxseeds
1¼ cups buckwheat flour
¼ cup old-fashioned rolled oats
2 tablespoons unsweetened coconut flakes
1 tablespoon baking powder
Pinch of sea salt
1 cup unsweetened, unflavored plant milk
½ cup unsweetened applesauce
¼ cup pure maple syrup
1 teaspoon pure vanilla extract
⅓ cup grain-sweetened, vegan mini chocolate chips
Sliced bananas, for serving

1. Place the flaxseeds in a small saucepan with ½ cup water. Cook over medium heat until the mixture gets a little sticky and appears stringy when it drips off a spoon, 3 to 4 minutes. Immediately strain the mixture into a glass measuring cup and set aside. Discard the seeds.

2. In a large bowl, whisk together the buckwheat flour, oats, coconut flakes, baking powder, and salt.

3. In a medium bowl, whisk together the milk, applesauce, maple syrup, vanilla, and 2 tablespoons of the reserved flax water.

4. Add the liquid mixture to the dry mixture and stir together to blend; the batter will be thick. Stir in the chocolate chips.

5. Heat a nonstick griddle over medium-low heat. Pour ⅓ cup batter for each pancake onto the griddle and spread gently. Cook for 6 to 8 minutes, until the pancakes look slightly dry

on top, are lightly browned on the bottom, and release easily from the pan. Flip and cook for about 5 minutes on the other side.

6. Repeat for the remaining batter, wiping off the griddle between batches. Serve hot with sliced bananas.

Storage: Place cooked pancakes in an airtight container and refrigerate for up to 5 days or freeze for up to 1 month. Reheat pancakes in a 350°F oven for 15 minutes for refrigerated pancakes or 25 minutes for frozen.

RECIPES

Savory Potato Pancakes

Makes 6 to 8 (4-inch) pancakes ■ *Ready in 30 minutes*

This recipe is a variation on a type of Indian pancake called childa, *made with chickpea flour and traditionally served with pickles, chutney, or even ketchup. These pancakes are delicious for breakfast, of course, but also for lunch or dinner; they travel well, too, so they make a good packed lunch.*

½ cup chickpea flour

½ cup oat flour

1 tablespoon nutritional yeast

1 teaspoon baking powder

¼ teaspoon baking soda

½ teaspoon onion powder

¼ teaspoon red pepper flakes (optional)

¼ teaspoon sea salt

¼ teaspoon freshly ground black pepper

1 cup unsweetened, unflavored plant milk or water

½ medium russet potato, finely grated (about ½ cup)

½ small leek, white and light green parts only, finely chopped (about ½ cup)

2 tablespoons finely chopped fresh cilantro

1 small garlic clove, minced (about ½ teaspoon)

1 tablespoon apple cider vinegar

2 teaspoons low-sodium tamari or soy sauce

Tomato Ketchup (page 237) or store-bought, or Cilantro Lime Chutney (page 239), for serving

1. In a large bowl, place the flours, nutritional yeast, baking powder, baking soda, onion powder, red pepper flakes (if using), and salt and pepper. Whisk together until well blended. Set aside.

2. In a medium bowl, place the milk, potato, leek, cilantro, garlic, vinegar, and tamari. Whisk to combine.

3. Create a well in the center of the dry mixture, and pour in the liquid mixture. Whisk gently to form a batter.

4. Heat a nonstick skillet over medium-low heat. For each pancake, pour about ⅓ cup batter into the skillet. Cook for 6 to 8 minutes, until the tops of the pancakes appear dry and the pancakes release easily from the pan.

5. Use a spatula to gently lift and flip the pancakes over. Cook for another 4 to 5 minutes, then remove to a warmed serving plate. Repeat with the remaining batter.

6. Serve hot with ketchup or chutney.

Storage: Store in an airtight container in the refrigerator for 3 to 4 days.

Spiced Apple Couscous

Makes about 6 cups ■ *Ready in 25 minutes*

This couscous dish makes a delicious warm breakfast, and it also tastes great chilled and served cold for lunch or as a snack. You can use another fruit in place of the apples; my other favorites are pears, mangoes, pineapples, and peaches.

1½ cups unsweetened, unflavored plant milk

¼ cup Date Paste (page 265)

1 teaspoon pure vanilla extract

1 cup whole wheat couscous

2 medium apples, cored and cut into ½-inch dice (about 2 cups)

½ cup unsweetened apple juice

¼ teaspoon ground cinnamon

¼ teaspoon ground cloves

2 tablespoons slivered or sliced almonds, for serving

1 tablespoon finely chopped fresh mint, for serving

1. In a medium saucepan, whisk together the milk, date paste, and vanilla. Bring to a boil over medium heat. Remove the pan from the heat, stir in the couscous, cover with a lid, and let stand until the liquid is absorbed, 5 to 10 minutes. Fluff with a fork.

2. Meanwhile, in a sauté pan, place the apples, apple juice, cinnamon, and cloves. Cook, uncovered, over medium heat, until softened, 5 to 10 minutes.

3. Add the cooked apples and any remaining juice to the couscous and mix well.

4. Serve warm or chill in the refrigerator and serve cold. Garnish with the almonds and fresh mint before serving.

Storage: Store in an airtight container in the refrigerator for 3 to 4 days.

RECIPES

Fig and Walnut Granola

Makes about 8 cups ■ Ready in 1½ hours

This granola stores beautifully and can be used in so many ways. It is good for breakfast, of course, especially with some fresh fruit and milk, and also as a snack, or as a topping on Peanut Butter Ice "Cream" (page 256). If the granola appears a bit moist at the end of an hour, don't worry; it will dry and get crisp once it is out of the oven and has cooled. You can replace the date paste with ¾ cup maple crystals or pure maple syrup.

4 cups old-fashioned rolled oats or any rolled grain flakes, such as barley, spelt, or rye

1 cup dried medium figs, trimmed and finely chopped

1 cup walnuts, finely chopped

2 tablespoons flaxseeds

¼ cup raisins

1 teaspoon ground cinnamon

¼ teaspoon ground allspice

2 pinches of sea salt

1 cup unsweetened applesauce

1 cup Date Paste (page 265)

1 teaspoon pure vanilla extract

1. Preheat the oven to 300°F. Line two rimmed baking sheets with parchment paper.

2. In a large bowl, place the oats, figs, walnuts, flaxseeds, raisins, cinnamon, allspice, and salt. Toss with your hands to mix.

3. In a small bowl, stir together the applesauce, date paste, and vanilla until well combined.

4. Add the applesauce mixture to the oats. Stir until thoroughly blended. Spread the oats evenly on the prepared baking sheets.

5. Bake until the mixture is dry, the oats are lightly browned, and the walnuts are crisp, 1 to 1¼ hours, stirring every 20 minutes. (The granola will crisp up after it cools.)

6. Remove from the oven and let cool on the baking sheets. As soon as the granola is completely cool, transfer to an airtight container.

Storage: Store in an airtight container at room temperature for 7 to 10 days.

RECIPES

Corn and Quinoa Baked Porridge

Makes 1 (8-inch square) porridge cake; about 6 cups ■ *Ready in 50 minutes*

*Baking sets this porridge into a lovely cake-like pudding topped with lightly
toasted seeds. If you are short on time, just skip the baking and serve the warm
porridge topped with the berries and seeds. It keeps well in the fridge for a few days.*

1 cup coarse cornmeal

3 cups unsweetened,
unflavored plant milk

1 cup dry quinoa, rinsed and
drained

¼ cup Date Paste (page 265)

1 teaspoon pure vanilla
extract

¼ teaspoon ground cinnamon

Pinch of sea salt

3 cups fresh or frozen berries

¼ cup pure maple syrup

¼ cup pumpkin seeds

¼ cup sunflower seeds

1. Preheat the oven to 350°F.

2. Pour 1 cup water into a small bowl. Whisk in the
   cornmeal and set aside.

3. In a medium saucepan, bring the milk to a boil
   over medium heat. Whisk in the quinoa, date
   paste, vanilla, cinnamon, and salt.

4. Whisking constantly, add the cornmeal and
   water. Bring to a simmer, then cover the pan
   and cook over low heat until the cornmeal and
   quinoa are almost cooked, 15 to 20 minutes,
   stirring frequently. (You can use a heat diffuser
   to keep the pan from overheating and the
   cornmeal from sticking to the bottom.) Remove
   from the heat and let stand for 5 to 10 minutes.

5. In a medium bowl, toss together the berries and
   maple syrup.

6. Spread half the cornmeal and quinoa mixture
   in an 8-inch square baking dish. Evenly spread
   the berries on top. Spoon the remaining mixture
   on top and gently spread to cover. Sprinkle with
   the pumpkin and sunflower seeds.

7. Bake in the oven for 20 minutes, until the seeds
   get a bit toasty and brown. Serve hot.

FORKS OVER KNIVES FAMILY

Sweet Potato Hash Brown Patties 🥖

Makes about 18 (2- to 3-inch) patties ■ *Ready in 50 minutes*

These baked hash brown patties make a very good school lunch—there's no need to reheat them. They can be eaten just as is or served with a tasty sauce.

2 tablespoons flaxseeds

2 pounds sweet potatoes (about 4 medium)

2 small zucchini (about ½ pound)

½ cup almond flour

½ cup oat or whole wheat flour

1 tablespoon garlic powder

1 tablespoon onion powder

½ cup finely chopped fresh parsley

⅓ cup fresh lime juice (from 2 limes)

½ teaspoon sea salt

¼ teaspoon freshly ground black pepper

Tahini Sauce (page 241), Tomato Ketchup (page 237) or store-bought, or Cilantro Lime Chutney (page 239), for topping or dipping (optional)

1. Preheat the oven to 400°F. Line two baking sheets with parchment paper.

2. Place the flaxseeds in a small saucepan with ¾ cup water. Cook over medium heat until the mixture gets a little sticky and appears stringy when it drips off a spoon, 3 to 4 minutes. Immediately strain the mixture into a glass measuring cup and set aside. Discard the seeds.

3. Using the large holes on a box grater, grate the unpeeled sweet potatoes; set aside. Grate the zucchini. Set aside.

4. In a large bowl, place the flours, garlic powder, onion powder, parsley, lime juice, and salt and pepper. Stir to combine.

5. Add the reserved sweet potatoes and zucchini and 3 tablespoons of the reserved flax water. Use a spatula or your hands to mix well. The mixture should be slightly moist and not too sticky; if it's dry, add more flax water, if it's too moist, add a bit more oat flour.

6. Place ⅓-cup scoops of the mixture on the prepared baking sheets. Press each mound into a patty about 2½ inches across and ½ inch high.

7. Bake until the tops of the patties are dry and the bottoms are brown and crisp, about 20 minutes.

8. Remove the baking sheets from the oven and let stand for 5 minutes. Then flip the patties over and bake for another 15 to 20 minutes, until the tops are lightly browned and crisp, and the patties are cooked through. Serve with tahini, ketchup, or chutney, if desired.

Storage: Let the patties cool to room temperature. Transfer them to an airtight container, and store in the refrigerator for 3 to 4 days.

RECIPES

Vegetable Breakfast Quesadillas

Makes 12 quesadillas ■ *Ready in 40 minutes*

Nothing beats a breakfast you can eat with your hands, and it's all the better when the dish is as versatile as this one. You can serve these quesadillas hot or cold, with guacamole and salsa or your kids' favorite dipping sauce, and for the more adventurous eaters, spice them up with some hot sauce. They are fantastic packed in a lunch, because they even taste great the day after they're made. And they make festive and delicious additions to a party spread or a picnic.

12 (10-inch) whole-grain wheat tortillas

6 cups White Bean Rosemary Dip (page 224; double the recipe)

1 large zucchini, thinly sliced (about 2 cups)

4 medium carrots, grated (about 2 cups)

3 lightly packed cups trimmed fresh spinach, finely chopped

1½ cups Green Pea Guacamole (page 231), for serving

1½ cups Sweet Salsa Fresca (page 229), for serving

1. Place a tortilla on a clean work surface. Evenly spread ½ cup white bean dip on one half of the tortilla.

2. Layer the zucchini, carrots, and spinach on top of the bean dip. Fold the other half over the vegetables and set aside. Repeat with the remaining tortillas, dip, and vegetables.

3. Preheat a nonstick griddle over medium heat. Toast the quesadillas on each side until crisp, slightly brown, and warmed through, about 5 minutes per side.

4. Cut the quesadillas in half using a pizza cutter.

5. Serve hot or cold, topped with guacamole and salsa.

Storage: Tightly wrap the quesadillas individually in wax paper and store in the refrigerator for up to 2 days.

Cauliflower and Potato Mash

Makes about 5 cups ■ *Ready in 45 minutes*

This is a hearty breakfast dish served, as it is here, on toast. The mash also makes a good filling for a burrito. If there are leftovers, stir in some cooked brown rice and sautéed greens and serve them for lunch.

1 medium onion, cut into ¼-inch dice (about 2 cups)

6 small garlic cloves, minced (about 1 tablespoon)

A ½-inch piece jalapeño pepper, stemmed, seeded, and finely chopped (optional)

1 tablespoon dried oregano

½ teaspoon ground turmeric

3 dried bay leaves

1 large potato (about ¾ pound), cut into ½-inch dice (about 3 cups)

½ medium cauliflower (about 1 pound), cored and cut into ½-inch florets (about 4 cups)

½ cup frozen edamame beans, rinsed and drained

1 medium tomato, cut into ½-inch pieces (about 1 cup)

4 scallions, white and green parts, thinly sliced (about 1 cup)

2 tablespoons fresh lime juice (from 1 lime)

Sea salt and freshly ground black pepper

10 slices whole-grain bread, toasted

2 tablespoons finely chopped fresh cilantro or parsley, for serving

1. In a large skillet, place the onion, garlic, jalapeño (if using), oregano, turmeric, bay leaves, and ¼ cup water. Cover and cook over medium-low heat, stirring once or twice, until the onion is translucent, about 10 minutes.

2. Stir in the potato and ¼ cup water. Cover and cook over medium heat for 5 minutes, until the potato is beginning to soften.

3. Add the cauliflower and stir to mix well. Cover and cook, stirring occasionally, for 10 minutes. Stir in the edamame. Cover and cook, stirring occasionally, for 5 to 10 minutes, until all the vegetables are tender but the edamame are still bright green. Add a little water as necessary to prevent sticking.

4. Add the tomato, scallions, lime juice, and salt and pepper to taste and heat through for a minute or two. Stir well. Remove and discard the bay leaves.

5. Serve over the whole-grain toast, garnished with the cilantro.

Fresh Fruit Muffins

Makes 12 muffins ■ *Ready in 1 hour*

This recipe is always yummy, no matter which fruit you use. It is fun to try different combinations of fruit puree or sauce and fresh fruits. Some of my favorite combinations are pureed oranges with chopped apples, pineapple puree with chopped pears, and mashed banana with fresh or frozen blueberries.

¾ cup unsweetened, unflavored plant milk

1 tablespoon ground flaxseed

1 teaspoon apple cider vinegar

¾ cup pure maple syrup

½ cup puree of any fresh fruit or unsweetened applesauce

1 teaspoon pure vanilla extract

1 cup unbleached all-purpose flour (see Note 1)

½ cup whole wheat flour

½ cup old-fashioned rolled oats

2 teaspoons baking powder

¼ teaspoon baking soda

2 pinches of sea salt

1 cup fresh or frozen berries or finely chopped fresh fruit (see Note 2)

1. Preheat the oven to 350°F. Line a standard muffin pan with cupcake liners or place a silicone muffin pan on a baking sheet.

2. In a medium bowl, combine the milk, ground flaxseed, and vinegar. Let stand for 5 to 10 minutes.

3. Add the maple syrup, fruit puree, and vanilla. Stir to blend well.

4. In large bowl, place the flours, oats, baking powder, baking soda, and salt. Whisk to blend. Add the liquid ingredients and gently stir just until combined. Add the fresh fruit and mix quickly and gently.

5. Divide the batter among the lined cups (about ⅓ cup each). Bake until a toothpick poked in the center of a muffin comes out dry, 30 to 45 minutes.

6. Remove the pan from the oven and place on a rack to cool for a few minutes. Unmold the muffins onto the rack. Serve warm or at room temperature.

Storage: Store in an airtight container in the refrigerator for 4 to 5 days.

Note 1: To make gluten-free muffins, replace the all-purpose flour with gluten-free oat flour, replace the whole wheat flour with sorghum flour, and make sure to use gluten-free rolled oats.

Note 2: If using very juicy fruit, such as peaches, cut it into bigger pieces and add to the batter after you have poured it into the muffin pan.

RECIPES

Zucchini Banana Walnut Muffins

Makes 12 muffins ■ Ready in 1 hour

These are perfect breakfast muffins. The addition of bananas makes them a little bit sweeter than traditional zucchini bread. Make a double batch and freeze the extras so that there are always quick grab-and-go breakfasts or snacks available.

1 cup unsweetened, unflavored plant milk

1 tablespoon ground flaxseed

1 teaspoon apple cider vinegar

3 ripe medium bananas, lightly mashed (about 1¼ cups)

1 medium zucchini, grated (about 1 cup)

¼ cup pure maple syrup

1 teaspoon pure vanilla extract

1 cup oat flour

1 cup whole wheat flour (see Note)

½ cup old-fashioned rolled oats

2 teaspoons baking powder

¼ teaspoon baking soda

2 pinches of sea salt

½ tablespoon poppy seeds

¼ cup chopped walnuts

1. Preheat the oven to 350°F. Line a standard muffin pan with cupcake liners or place a silicone muffin pan on a baking sheet.

2. In a medium bowl, stir together the milk, ground flaxseed, and vinegar. Let stand for 5 to 10 minutes.

3. Add the bananas to the milk along with the zucchini, maple syrup, and vanilla. Stir until well blended.

4. In large bowl, whisk together the flours, oats, baking powder, baking soda, and salt. Add the poppy seeds and walnuts, and mix well.

5. Add the banana-zucchini mixture to the dry ingredients. Mix quickly and gently just until combined.

6. Evenly divide the batter among the lined cups (it'll be a little over ⅓ cup each). Bake in the oven until a toothpick inserted in the center of a muffin comes out dry, 40 to 45 minutes.

7. Remove the pan from the oven and place on a rack to cool for a few minutes. Unmold the muffins onto the rack to cool completely. Serve.

Storage: Store in an airtight container at room temperature for up to 1 day or place in a re-sealable bag and freeze for up to 1 month.

Note: To make these gluten-free, replace the whole wheat flour with sorghum flour and make sure to use gluten-free oat flour and rolled oats.

RECIPES

SNACKS

Herbed Popcorn

Makes about 2 cups popcorn kernels, enough for 10 quarts popcorn ■ *Ready in 45 minutes (plus cooling and popping time)*

Family movie night practically demands a big bowl of popcorn, but it can be hard to get tasty flavorings to stick to oil-free, air-popped kernels. Some recipes call for spraying or sprinkling the popcorn with tamari or Bragg's Amino, but that leaves you with soggy popcorn. The answer is to apply the seasoning before *air popping. This method is especially useful because it allows you to preseason a large amount of popping corn so that it's ready for you to pop whenever the urge strikes for a bowl of the crunchy good stuff.*

2 tablespoons white wine vinegar

1 tablespoon finely chopped fresh rosemary

1 tablespoon finely chopped fresh thyme

Sea salt and freshly ground black pepper

2 cups popcorn kernels

1. Preheat the oven to 250°F. Line a rimmed baking sheet with parchment paper.

2. In a medium bowl, stir together the vinegar, rosemary, thyme, and salt and pepper to taste. Let stand for 5 minutes.

3. Add the popcorn kernels and stir until well coated. Let stand for 10 minutes.

4. Spread the corn on the prepared baking sheet and bake until completely dry, about 30 minutes. Let cool completely.

5. Place the kernels in a colander and shake gently to separate the dried spices that might have settled at the bottom of the baking sheet (this will keep the dried spices from burning in the air popper).

6. To use, pop in an electric or microwave air popper as desired; ½ cup kernels will yield about 10 cups popcorn.

Storage: Store the seasoned kernels in an airtight container at room temperature for up to 1 month.

Nachos 📷

Makes 1 (9 × 13-inch) pan; about 4 cups chips ■ *Ready in 50 minutes*

Nachos are a favorite with adults and kids alike, no doubt due to the satisfyingly contrasting flavors and textures of the crunchy chips, creamy cheese, bracing pico de gallo, and filling beans. It is not easy to find good oil-free and salt-free tortilla chips in most stores. Good thing it's so quick and easy is to make them yourself!

8 corn tortillas, each cut into 6 triangles

1 (15-ounce) can pinto or black beans, rinsed and drained (about 1½ cups)

1 cup Pico de Gallo (page 230)

2 cups Nacho Cheese (page 232)

2 scallions, white and green parts, thinly sliced (about ½ cup)

¼ cup sliced olives (optional)

1. Preheat the oven to 350°F. Line two baking sheets with parchment paper.

2. Spread the tortilla triangles on the prepared baking sheets, making sure not to layer the chips on top of one another or they will not get crisp. Bake in the oven for 20 minutes, until crisp.

3. Transfer the chips to a 9 × 13-inch baking dish. Top with the beans, pico de gallo, and cheese. Bake just until the cheese is hot and lightly browned, about 15 minutes.

4. Garnish with scallions and olives (if using). Serve at once.

Storage: If you've made a lot of chips, let them cool on the baking sheet, then transfer them to an airtight container and store for up to 7 days.

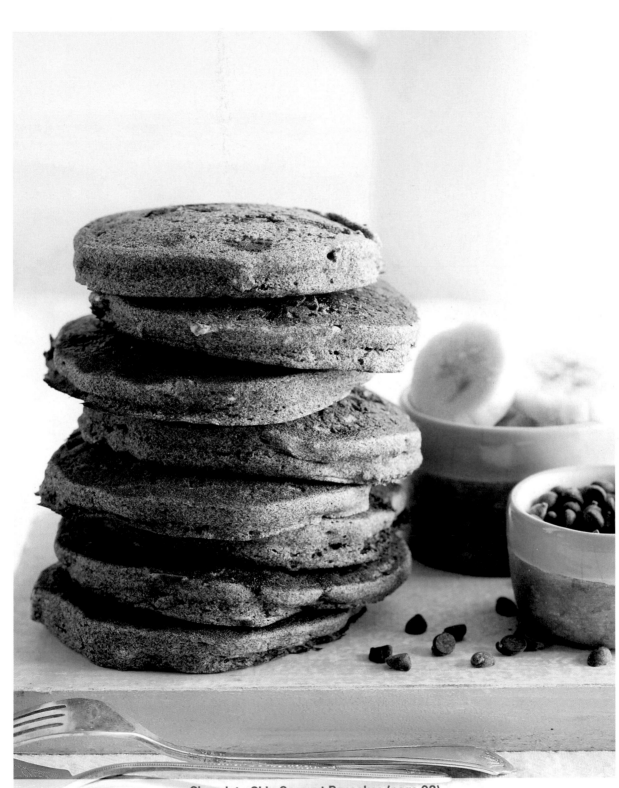

Chocolate Chip Coconut Pancakes (page 92)

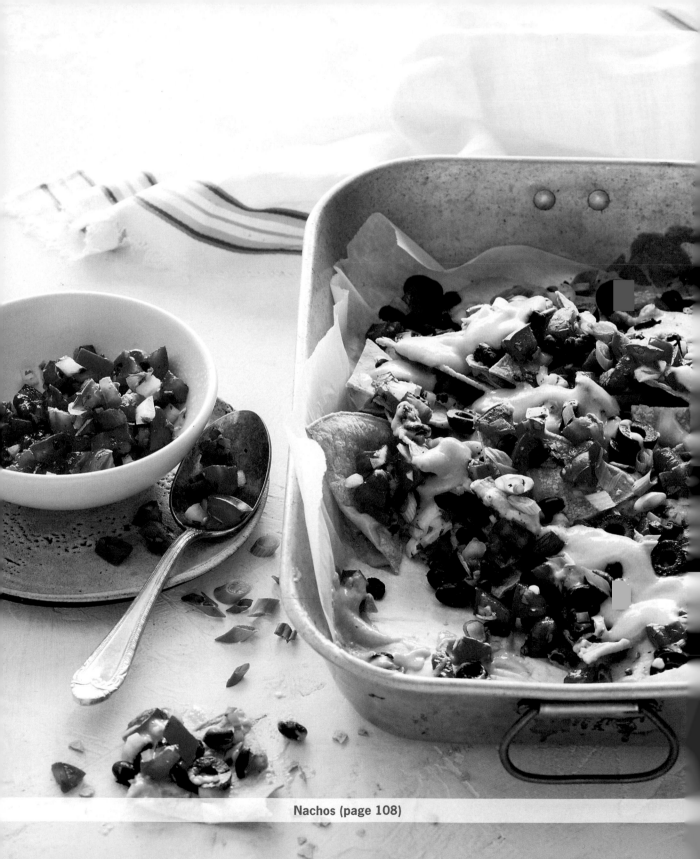

Nachos (page 108)

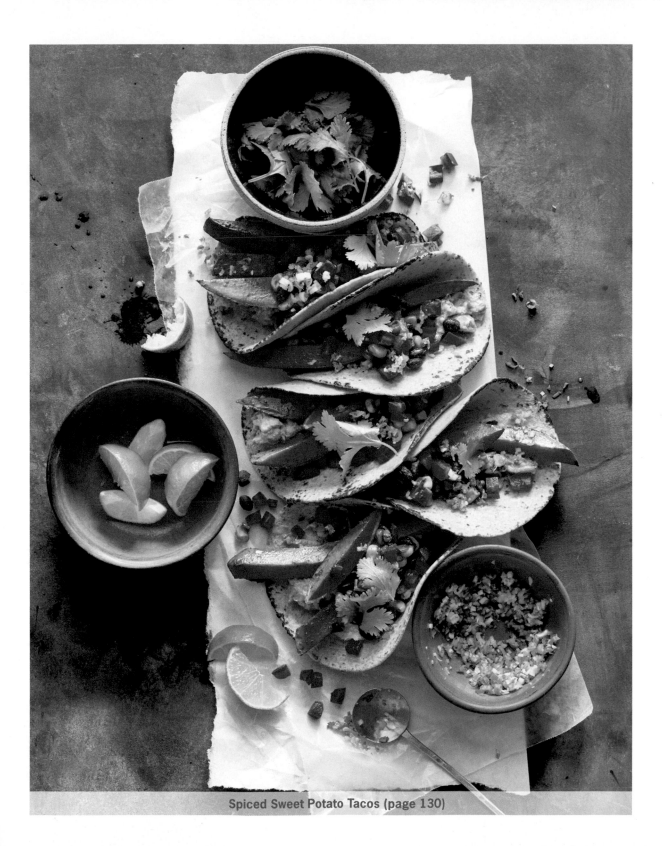

Spiced Sweet Potato Tacos (page 130)

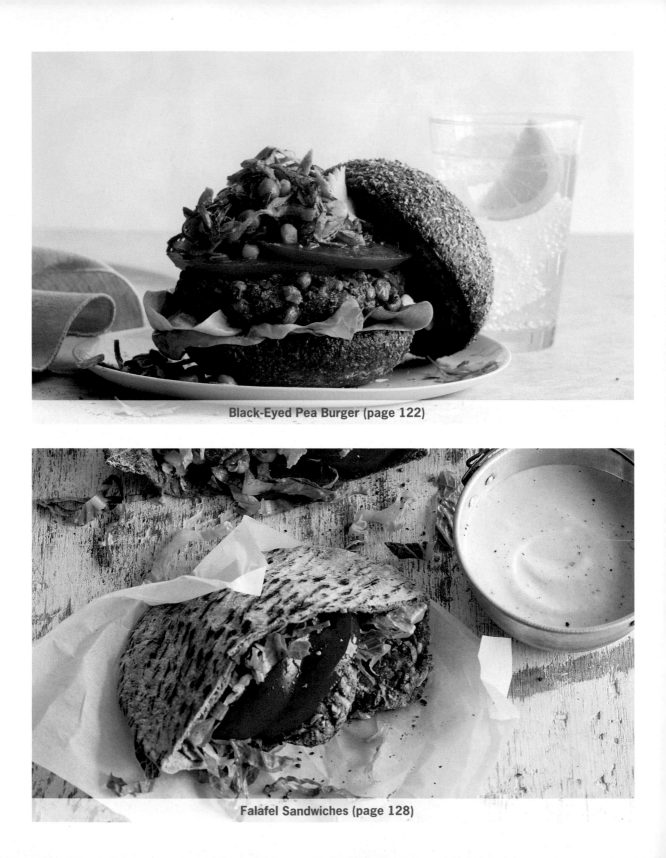

Black-Eyed Pea Burger (page 122)

Falafel Sandwiches (page 128)

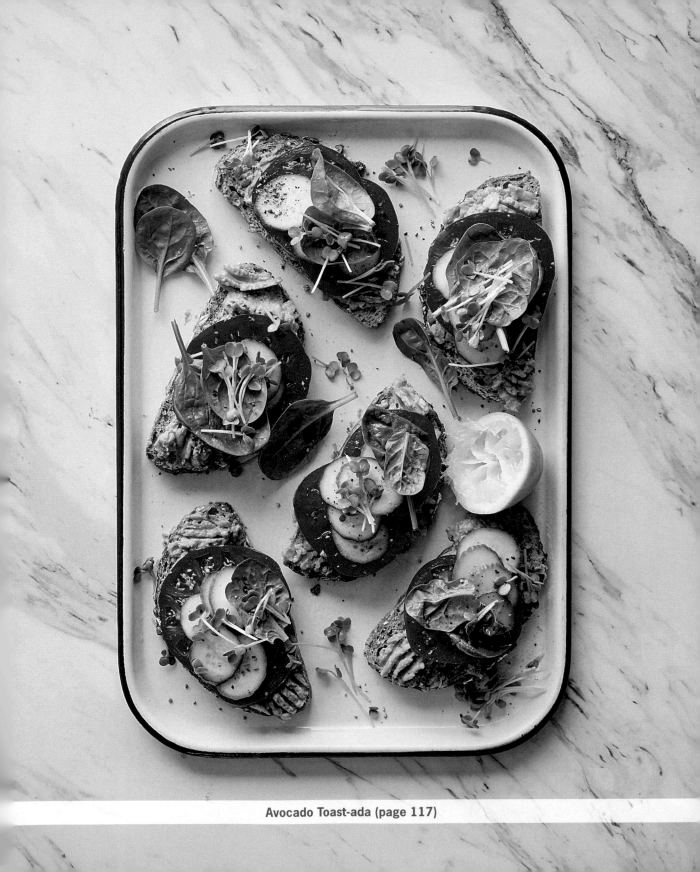

Avocado Toast-ada (page 117)

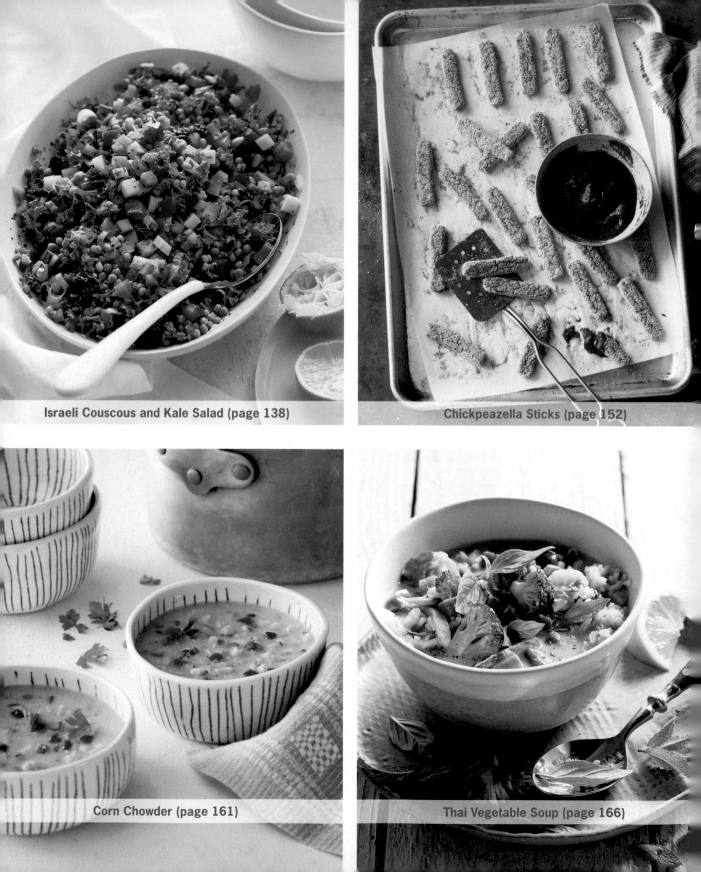

Israeli Couscous and Kale Salad (page 138)

Chickpeazella Sticks (page 152)

Corn Chowder (page 161)

Thai Vegetable Soup (page 166)

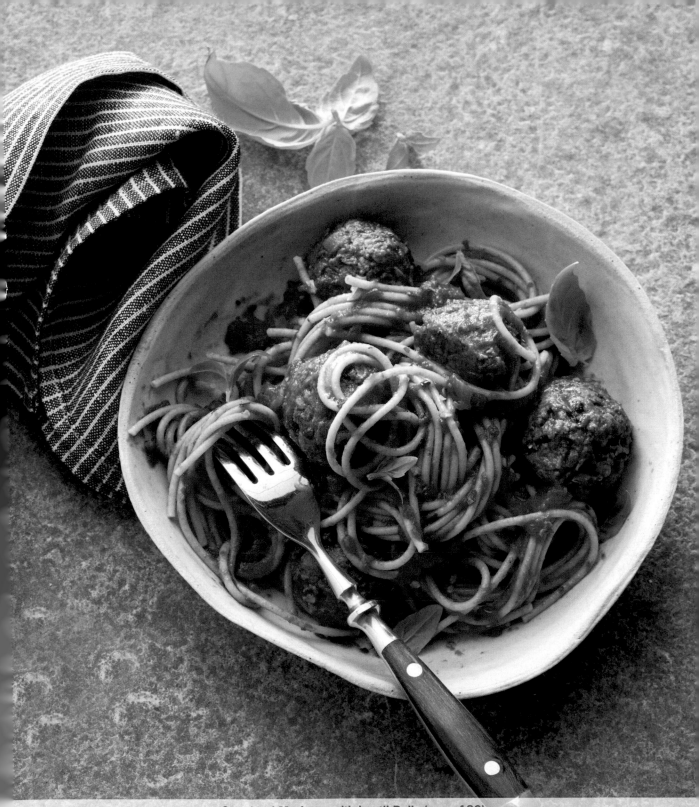

Spaghetti Marinara with Lentil Balls (page 186)

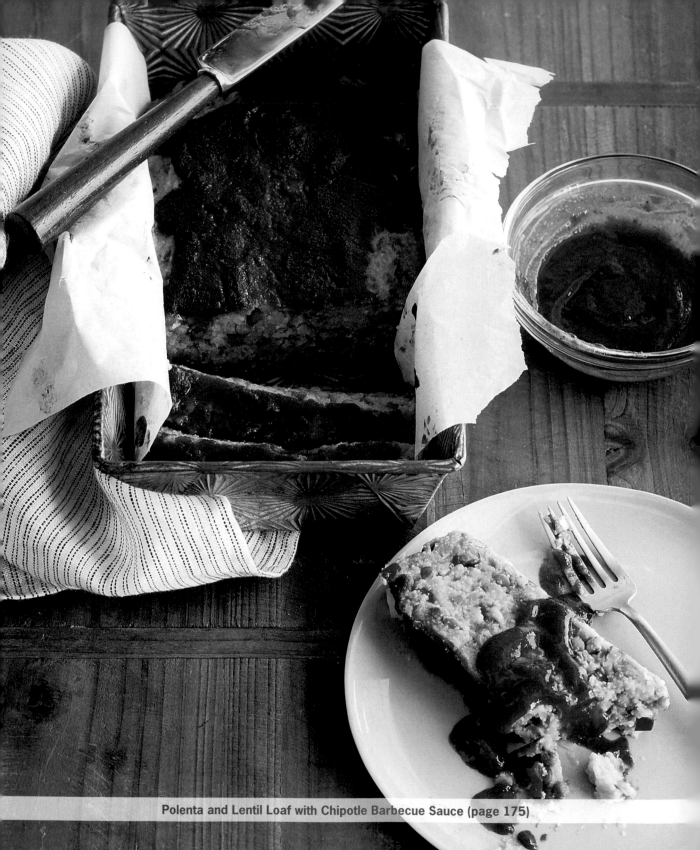

Polenta and Lentil Loaf with Chipotle Barbecue Sauce (page 175)

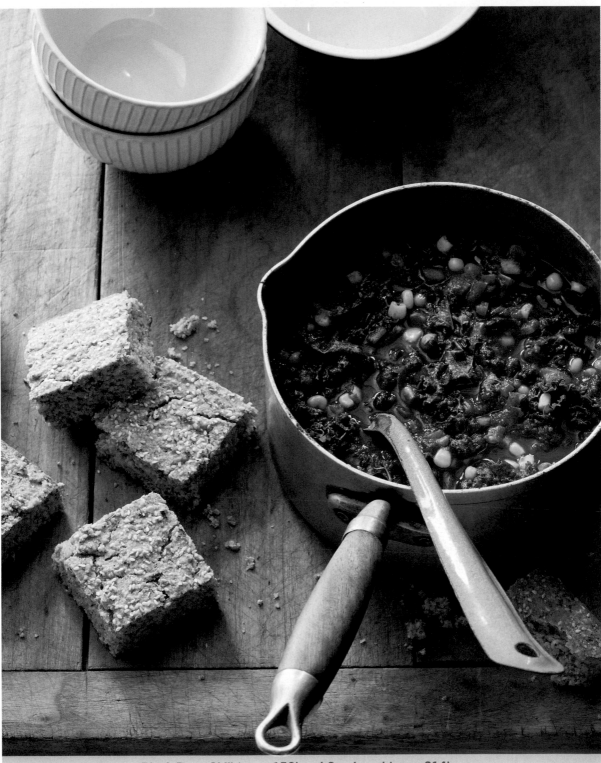

Black Bean Chili (page 158) and Cornbread (page 214)

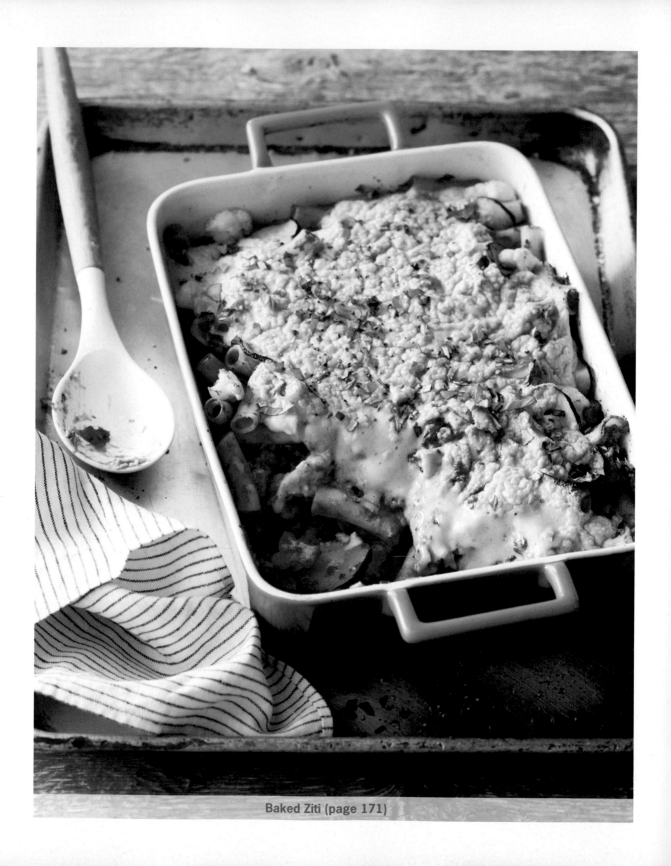

Baked Ziti (page 171)

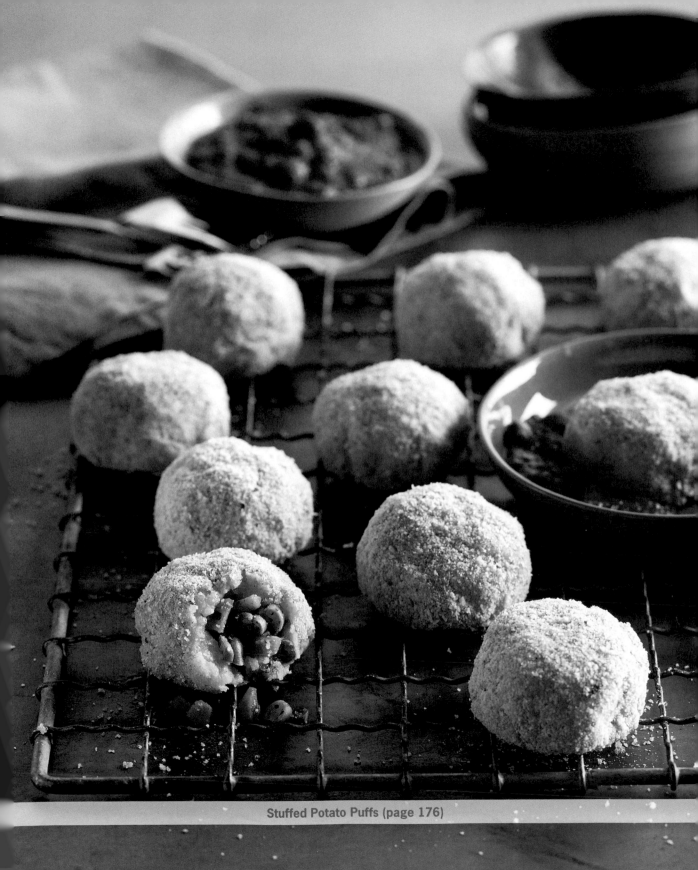

Stuffed Potato Puffs (page 176)

Mexican Bowl (page 200), Couscous Bowl (page 199), and Tokyo Bowl (page 202)

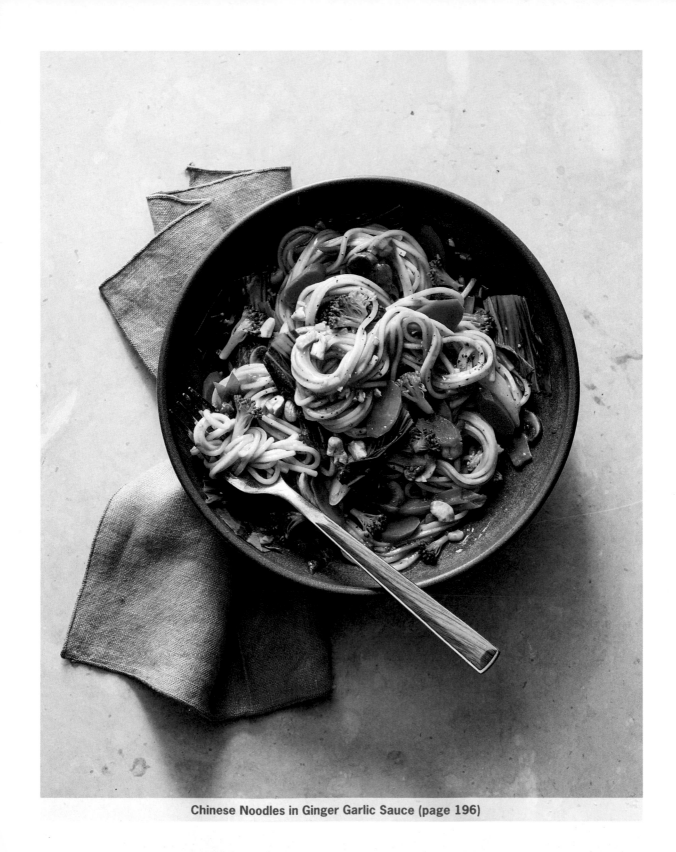

Chinese Noodles in Ginger Garlic Sauce (page 196)

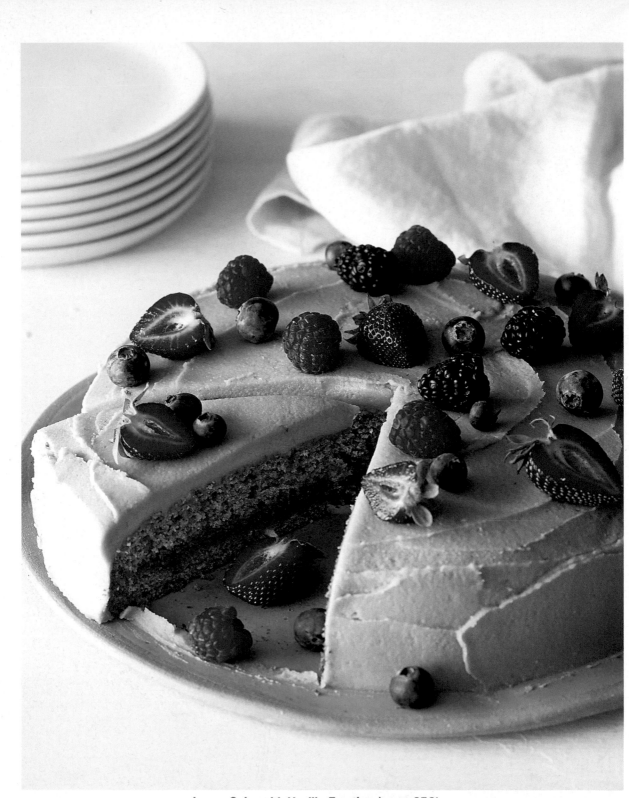

Layer Cake with Vanilla Frosting (page 252)

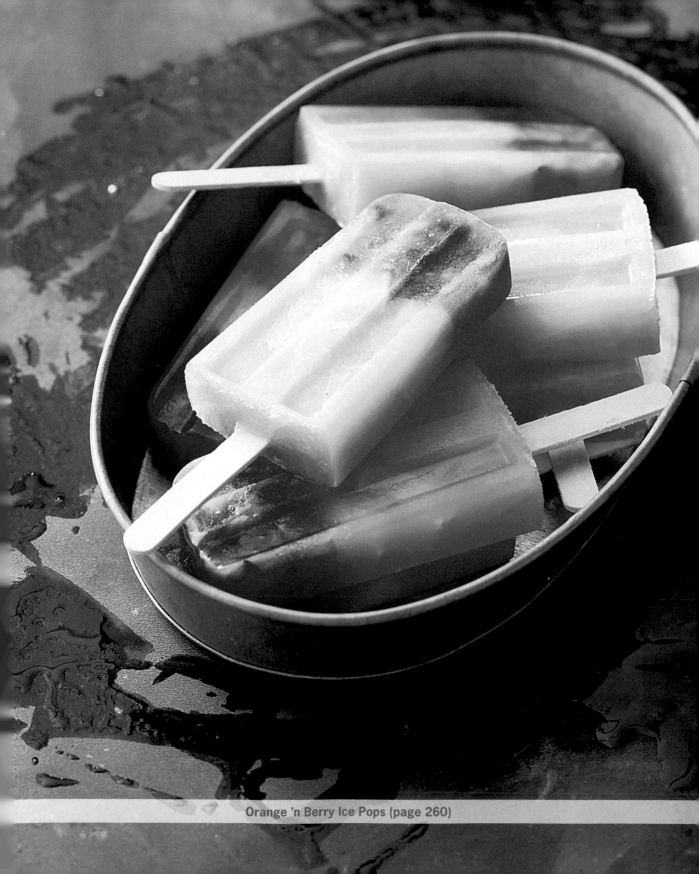

Orange 'n Berry Ice Pops (page 260)

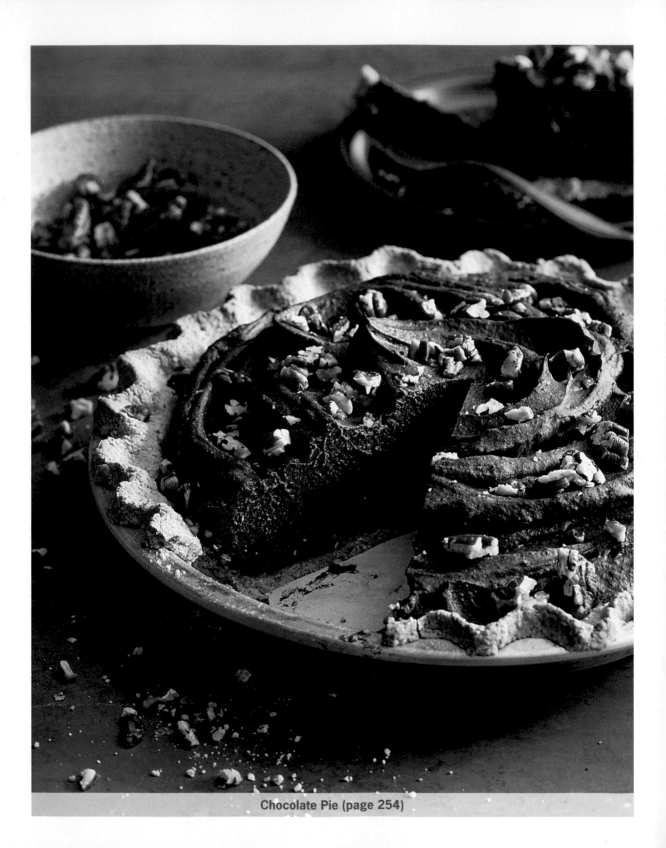

Chocolate Pie (page 254)

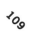

Chocolate Bliss Balls

Makes about 30 (1-inch) balls ■ *Ready in 40 minutes*

These yummy chocolate treats are ready in minutes and they're great for potlucks, picnics, and kids' parties. Better still, they will keep in the fridge for a week, so you can make a batch and have them around for those moments when only a rich, chocolate bite will do! For best results, use good-quality cocoa.

½ cup unsalted pumpkin seeds

½ cup unsalted sunflower seeds

2 cups old-fashioned rolled oats

¾ cup natural unsweetened cocoa powder

1 teaspoon pure vanilla extract

2 pinches of sea salt (optional)

¾ cup Date Paste (page 265)

1. In a food processor, pulse the seeds until coarsely chopped. Remove ¼ cup of the mixture and set aside on a small plate.
2. Add the oats, cocoa powder, vanilla, and salt (if using) to the food processor. Pulse the mixture until the oats are almost pulverized.
3. Add the date paste and pulse until the mixture starts to bind together, adding 1 or 2 tablespoons water as necessary to help it bind.
4. Scoop out 1 tablespoon of the mixture and roll into a 1-inch ball. Coat all over with the reserved ground seeds. Repeat with the rest of the cocoa mixture and ground seeds.

Storage: Store in an airtight container in the refrigerator for up to 1 week.

RECIPES

Nut-Stuffed Dates

Makes 20 stuffed dates ■ *Ready in 10 minutes*

This is a nice snack for before or after exercise or hikes. These dates travel well so they're good to bring to the beach and on picnics. You can use dried figs or apricots in place of the dates, and replace the almonds and pistachios with cashews, walnuts, or pecans.

20 pitted jumbo dates, slit open

¼ cup unsalted roasted almonds

¼ cup shelled unsalted pistachios

Stuff each date with a few almonds and/or pistachios.

Storage: Store in an airtight container in the refrigerator for up to 1 week.

Chickpea and Cucumber Salad

Makes about 3 cups ■ *Ready in 10 minutes*

This salad can be pulled together in minutes, and is perfect to munch on while doing homework or watching TV. For a bigger salad, add more vegetables. Jícama, tomatoes, carrots, and celery are particularly good additions here.

1 (15-ounce) can chickpeas, rinsed and drained (about 1½ cups)

1 medium cucumber, cut into 1-inch dice (about 1½ cups)

Juice from 1 lemon (about 2 tablespoons)

Pinch of sweet or mild paprika

2 or 3 fresh mint leaves, finely chopped

Sea salt (optional)

1. In a medium bowl, mix the chickpeas, cucumber, lemon juice, paprika, mint leaves, and salt (if using).
2. Serve at once or chill before serving.

Storage: Store in an airtight container in the refrigerator for 2 to 3 days.

Tropical Fruit and Berry Smoothie

Makes about 4 cups ■ *Ready in 5 minutes*

*Smoothies can be a great, quick pick-me-up snack. And they can be a
boon for the parents of active, lean kids who are often too busy to eat
(see page 40). The tropical flavors of mangoes and pineapples combined
with the sweet berries are especially nutritious and satisfying.*

**2 cups cold water or
unflavored, unsweetened
plant milk**

**2 lightly packed cups trimmed
fresh spinach**

1½ cups frozen mango pieces

**1½ cups frozen pineapple
pieces**

1 cup fresh or frozen berries

In a blender, in batches if necessary, place the
water, spinach, mango, pineapple, and berries.
Blend until smooth. Serve at once.

Fresh Fruit "Mince" on Romaine Leaves

Makes 4 to 6 rolls; about 2 cups filling ■ *Ready in 5 minutes*

Serve this fresh and tasty combination of minced fruits rolled up in romaine or kale leaves, or scoop up the filling using baked corn or toasted pita chips. It's also good spooned over cooked oatmeal.

1 medium apple, cored and finely chopped (about 1 cup)

1 large pear, cored and finely chopped (about 1¼ cups)

¼ cup Date Paste (page 265)

1 teaspoon grated lemon zest (optional)

4 to 6 romaine lettuce leaves

1. In a medium bowl, stir together the apple, pear, date paste, and lemon zest (if using).

2. To serve, place a few spoonfuls of the mince onto each romaine leaf and roll up.

Storage: Store the filling in an airtight container in the refrigerator for 3 to 4 days.

Seasoned Corn on the Cob

Makes 6 ears of corn ■ Ready in 20 minutes

Fresh corn on the cob makes a great quick snack because it doesn't really need much seasoning or extended cooking. Just a little flavor enhancing makes it more fun. These make a good packed lunch, too.

1 to 2 teaspoons Italian seasoning or sweet or mild paprika

1 teaspoon garlic powder

6 fresh ears of corn, shucked

1 lemon, cut into 6 wedges

1. In a small bowl, mix the Italian seasoning and garlic powder. Set aside.

2. You can fire-roast or boil the corn. *To fire-roast,* turn a gas burner on medium-high and place the corn directly against the flame. Use tongs to turn the ears occasionally until they are lightly browned all over. *To boil,* bring a large pot of water to a boil over high heat. Add the corn and cook for 5 to 7 minutes. Drain thoroughly.

3. Dip 1 lemon wedge in the spice mixture, then squeeze and rub it over 1 ear of corn so that the spice mixture and juice together coat the kernels. Repeat with the remaining spice mixture, lemon wedges, and corn. Serve warm.

Storage: Store leftovers in an airtight container in the refrigerator for up to 2 days.

FORKS OVER KNIVES FAMILY

Crispy Vegetables

Makes 4 cups ▪ Ready in 15 minutes

A great way to start off the week is to very lightly boil vegetables and shock them in ice water. This preserves their bright color and crispness, making them tastier for kids. They can be stored in the refrigerator for several days and served by the handful either alone or with a dipping sauce.

4 cups trimmed green beans, sugar snap peas; snow peas; or broccoli or cauliflower florets, cut into 1-inch pieces

Sea salt

Dipping sauce, for serving (optional)

1. Bring a large pot of lightly salted water to a boil over high heat. Prepare a large bowl of ice water.

2. Add the vegetables to the boiling water and cook for about 1 minute, until brightly colored and very lightly softened (they should still be very crisp).

3. Drain and immediately plunge the vegetables into the ice water. Let stand until completely cool.

4. Drain thoroughly and serve alone or with a dipping sauce.

Storage: Store in an airtight container in the refrigerator for up to 4 days.

Peanut Butter, Banana, and Crushed Berry Sandwiches

Makes 4 sandwiches ■ Ready in 20 minutes

This takes an ordinary PB&J sandwich and steps it up several notches by replacing the jelly with fresh bananas and crushed berries. If it's not berry season, substitute thinly sliced pears or apples, or stone fruits like peaches and plums. If using harder fruits such as apples or pears, add ¼ cup water when cooking. No matter what fruit you use, these sandwiches are great not only for a quick pick-me-up snack but also in packed lunches.

1½ cups fresh or defrosted frozen berries (any variety)

8 slices whole-grain bread, toasted

4 tablespoons unsalted natural peanut butter

2 ripe medium bananas, thinly sliced

1. Place the berries in a small saucepan and crush them lightly with the back of a spoon. Cook over medium-low heat until they are soft, 3 to 4 minutes. Remove from the heat and let cool.

2. Spread 1 slice of the whole-grain toast with 1 tablespoon of the peanut butter. Repeat with 3 more toasts. Arrange the banana slices on top, overlapping them slightly to cover the peanut butter.

3. Spread the cooled crushed fruit on top of the bananas, dividing it evenly among the 4 toasts. Top each with one of the remaining 4 toasts.

4. Cut the sandwiches in half, if desired. Serve at once or wrap tightly and refrigerate until ready to serve.

Storage: Tightly wrap the sandwiches individually in wax paper and store in the refrigerator for up to 2 days.

Avocado Toast-ada 🔖 📷

Makes 6 toast-adas ▪ Ready in 15 minutes

This is one of my favorite snacks. Personally, I don't think it requires any dressing beyond the lemon juice, but for a little extra flourish you can drizzle some Tahini Sauce (page 241) on top.

1 Hass avocado, pitted and peeled

6 slices whole-grain bread, toasted

2 ripe medium tomatoes, thinly sliced (about 2 cups)

1 medium cucumber, thinly sliced (about 1½ cups)

1 to 2 cups baby romaine or spinach leaves

½ to ⅔ cup fresh alfalfa sprouts (optional)

Sea salt and freshly ground black pepper

Juice of 1 lemon (about 2 tablespoons)

1. Slice the avocado into 6 wedges and use a table knife or spoon to spread one wedge on each slice of whole-grain toast.
2. On top of the avocado, layer the tomato and cucumber slices and the romaine leaves. Pile the sprouts (if using) on top. Season with salt and pepper to taste and sprinkle with the lemon juice. Serve at once.

Storage: Tightly wrap the toast-adas individually in wax paper and store in the refrigerator for up to 1 day.

RECIPES

WRAPS, ROLL-UPS, AND BURGERS

Buckwheat Sloppy Joes on Toast

Makes about 8 cups (about 5 dozen little toasts or 8 sloppy joes) ■ Ready in 45 minutes

If you're looking for a less messy way to enjoy sloppy joes, try serving smaller spoonfuls of the mixture on small pieces of toasted bread, as in this recipe. In fact, you can even serve them as an appetizer this way. But if you (or your kids) prefer the traditional way, as fun, messy— and delicious!—as it can be, then serve them on burger buns.

½ cup dried red lentils

1 leek, white and light green parts only, finely chopped (about ½ cup)

1 small onion, minced (about 1 cup)

4 ounces button mushrooms, trimmed and cut into ¼-inch dice (about 1½ cups)

1 green bell pepper, cored, seeded, and cut into ¼-inch dice (about 1 cup)

12 small garlic cloves, minced (about 2 tablespoons)

1 (6-ounce) can no-salt-added tomato paste

2 tablespoons red wine vinegar

1 tablespoon Date Paste (page 265)

1 tablespoon mild white miso

1. Soak the lentils in 1 cup water for 20 minutes. Drain.

2. In a large saucepan, place the drained lentils, the leek, onion, mushrooms, green bell pepper, garlic, and 1 cup water. Cover the pan and cook over medium heat for 10 minutes, or until the onion is translucent.

3. Meanwhile, in a medium bowl, place the tomato paste, vinegar, date paste, miso, Worcestershire sauce, tamari, paprika, and 2 cups water. Whisk into a paste.

4. Add the paste to the lentil and vegetable mixture along with the buckwheat, tomatoes, red bell pepper, and salt and pepper to taste. Cover and cook over medium-low heat, stirring occasionally, for 15 to 20 minutes, or until the buckwheat is completely cooked and the liquid

RECIPES

1 tablespoon vegan Worcestershire sauce

1 tablespoon low-sodium tamari or soy sauce

1 tablespoon sweet or mild paprika

1 cup whole buckwheat groats

4 Roma (plum) tomatoes, cut into ¼-inch dice (about 2 cups)

1 red bell pepper, cored, seeded, and cut into ¼-inch dice (about 1 cup)

Sea salt and freshly ground black pepper

16 slices whole-grain bread, or 8 whole-grain burger buns, for serving

2 scallions, white and green parts, thinly sliced (about ½ cup), for serving

2 tablespoons finely chopped fresh cilantro or parsley, for serving (optional)

is absorbed. Add water if necessary to keep the mixture from sticking.

5. Meanwhile, preheat the oven to 350°F. Cut each slice of bread into 4 squares. Spread them out on a baking sheet and toast in the oven for 10 minutes. Turn them over and toast for another 10 minutes, or until lightly brown. (Alternatively, toast the buns in the oven until lightly browned.)

6. Pour a spoonful of the sloppy joe filling onto each bread square. Garnish with the scallions and cilantro (if using). (Alternatively, spoon the sloppy joe mixture onto the bottom halves of the burger buns; garnish if desired and top with the other half of the bun.) Serve hot.

Potato-bello Burritos

Makes 10 burritos ■ *Ready in 1 hour*

The lightly smoky taste of this potato-and-mushroom filling combines with the cumin-spiced beans, rice, and pico de gallo to create pleasing layers of distinct flavor and aroma. Ground ancho and pasilla chiles are chile powders well worth seeking out for their mild heat and lovely fruity flavor. They can be found in the Hispanic aisle of a well-stocked grocery store or in Hispanic markets. If you can't find them, substitute good-quality chili powder.

FOR THE POTATO-BELLO FILLING

1 medium red onion, cut into ½-inch dice (about 2 cups)

2 portobello mushrooms, stemmed and cut into ½-inch-thick strips (about 3 cups)

6 to 8 small garlic cloves, minced (3 to 4 teaspoons)

1 medium Yukon Gold potato (about ½ pound), cut into ½-inch dice (about 2 cups)

1 red bell pepper, cored, seeded, and cut into ½-inch dice (about 1 cup)

1 teaspoon smoked paprika

2 teaspoons dried Mexican oregano

1 bunch Swiss chard, stems discarded, leaves roughly chopped (about 4 cups)

Sea salt and freshly ground black pepper

1. Make the filling: In a large sauté pan, add the onion, mushrooms, garlic, and ¼ cup water. Cook over medium heat, covered, until the onion begins to turn translucent, about 5 minutes.

2. Add the potato, bell pepper, paprika, and oregano. Cover and cook until the potato is almost tender, about 15 minutes.

3. Add the chard and salt and pepper to taste, and cook until the greens have wilted and the potato is completely cooked, about 5 minutes. Set aside.

4. Assemble the burritos: Warm a tortilla for about 20 seconds on each side in a dry skillet set over medium heat. Or if you have a gas stove, place a tortilla straight over the flame for a few seconds on each side. Cover with a large damp cloth. Repeat with the remaining tortillas. Keep them covered until ready to use.

FOR THE BURRITOS

10 (10-inch) whole wheat
  tortillas

Black Bean Spread
  (page 226), warmed

3 cups cooked brown rice,
  warmed

1 small head romaine lettuce,
  shredded (about 4 cups)

Pico de Gallo (page 230)

5. Prepare a work station: Arrange the tortillas, bean spread, filling, rice, lettuce, and about 2 cups of the pico de gallo alongside one another.

6. Place 1 warmed tortilla on a plate. Place about ¼ cup of the bean spread in the center of the tortilla, flattening the beans slightly and leaving at least 2 inches of the tortilla uncovered along the edge. Top with about ½ cup filling and ¼ cup rice. Top with lettuce and about 2 tablespoons pico de gallo.

7. Fold in the left and right sides of the tortilla, and then fold up the bottom to cover the filling. Roll the tortilla away from you while securing the two sides that have been folded in. Place the tortilla seam side down on a serving platter. Repeat with the remaining tortillas and filling. These are best served warm, with the remaining pico de gallo.

Storage: If you must wait a little bit before serving, individually wrap the burritos tightly in wax paper until ready to serve, or refrigerate for up to 2 days. This ensures that they will hold together better when served later.

RECIPES

Black-Eyed Pea Burgers 🥡 📷

Makes 6 burgers ■ *Ready in 1½ hours*

The flavor of this burger was inspired by Creole spices, and it's especially tasty served with Red Cabbage Coleslaw (page 144) on top. To get ahead, you can make the burger mix the day before, and bake the burgers the day of serving. They freeze well, so make a double batch and freeze half.

1 medium Yukon Gold potato (about ½ pound), chopped (about 2 cups)

½ red bell pepper, chopped (about ½ cup)

2 small celery stalks, chopped (about ½ cup)

½ small onion, chopped (about ½ cup)

2 small garlic cloves, chopped (about 1 teaspoon)

2½ tablespoons Mild Creole Seasoning (page 169) or store-bought

⅛ teaspoon cayenne pepper (optional)

1 (15-ounce) can black-eyed peas, rinsed and drained (about 1½ cups)

4 scallions, white and green parts, thinly sliced (about 1 cup)

¼ cup chopped fresh parsley

¼ teaspoon sea salt

¼ teaspoon freshly ground black pepper

3 tablespoons arrowroot powder

6 whole wheat burger buns, toasted

1. In a food processor, place the potato, bell pepper, celery, onion, and garlic. Pulse until finely chopped, scraping down the sides once or twice.

2. Transfer to a large nonstick skillet (or place a skillet or a flame diffuser under a regular skillet to prevent sticking). Add the Creole seasoning and the cayenne (if using). Cook over medium-low heat, stirring often, until all the liquid from the vegetables has evaporated, 7 to 10 minutes.

3. Add the black-eyed peas, scallions, parsley, and salt and pepper. Mix well and cook, stirring occasionally, until the flavors have blended and the moisture has evaporated, 7 to 10 minutes.

4. Remove from the heat and use a potato masher or wooden spoon to coarsely mash the black-eyed peas. Avoid completely mashing the peas; you want some texture. Transfer the mixture to a baking sheet and set aside until completely cool.

5. Sprinkle the arrowroot powder over the cooled mixture and use your hands to gently work it in. (If desired, cover and store the mixture in the refrigerator for 1 day.)

Lettuce leaves, for serving

1 large tomato, thinly sliced, for serving

Red Cabbage Coleslaw (page 144; optional), for serving

Mustard, for serving

Tomato Ketchup (page 237) or store-bought, for serving

6. When ready to form and bake the patties, preheat the oven to 400°F. Line a baking sheet with parchment paper.

7. Scoop out about ⅓ cup of the mixture. Form into a 2½- to 3-inch patty and place it on the prepared baking sheet. Repeat with the remaining mixture to make 6 patties total.

8. Bake about 25 minutes, or until the top of the burgers are firm and crisp. Flip the burgers over using a thin spatula and bake until cooked through and lightly browned, 20 to 25 minutes more.

9. Serve the burgers in toasted burger buns with lettuce, tomato slices, coleslaw (if using), mustard, and ketchup.

Storage: Formed and unbaked patties can be frozen on the baking sheet. Once frozen, wrap tightly and store in the freezer for up to 1 month. Bake from frozen, adding about 10 minutes onto the baking time. To store burgers in the buns for lunches, wrap them individually in wax paper and store in the refrigerator for up to 2 days.

RECIPES

Fresh Vegetable Temaki Rolls

Makes 10 rolls ▪ *Ready in 1 hour*

With creamy avocado and nutty roasted sesame seeds, these bright temaki rolls really don't need any dipping sauce, but if your crew loves to dip, you can serve the rolls with Tamari Sesame Dipping Sauce (page 228). It can speed things up to grate the carrot and daikon radish in the food processor. These temaki rolls are good for a packed lunch.

3 cups cooked short-grain brown rice (from about 1 cup dry)

1 tablespoon roasted sesame seeds (any kind)

1 tablespoon brown rice vinegar

1 teaspoon low-sodium tamari or soy sauce

5 nori sheets

2 Hass avocados, peeled, pitted, and each sliced into 10 to 15 thin wedges

1 medium cucumber, cut into thin 2½-inch-long strips (about 2 cups)

2 medium carrots, grated (about 1 cup)

½ daikon radish, peeled and grated (about 1 cup)

2 scallions, white and green parts, thinly sliced (about ½ cup)

1. In a large bowl, place the rice, sesame seeds, vinegar, and tamari and mix well.

2. Prepare an assembly station: on a clean work surface, have ready the nori sheets, the rice stuffing, the avocados, cucumber, carrots, radish, and scallions, and a small dish of water.

3. Heat a large skillet over medium heat until hot. Working with one at a time, toast the nori sheets in the skillet for 30 to 45 seconds. Fold each sheet in half; it will easily break into two even rectangles.

4. Place one of the rectangles on a cutting board or clean kitchen towel with the long side parallel to you. Spread about ¼ cup of rice on the left side of the rectangle, filling ⅓ to ½ of the sheet and leaving about ½ inch of space in the lower left-hand corner.

5. Top the rice with 2 or 3 avocado wedges. Top with some of the cucumber, carrots, radish, and scallions, arranging them diagonally from the

upper left-hand corner to the bottom right-hand corner of the rice.

6. Fold the left bottom corner of the rectangle up toward the top right-hand corner of the rice to cover the fillings. Tuck it under the rice and continue to roll the rectangle in the same direction to form a tight cone shape. Use a small brush or your fingertips to wet the exposed corner of the rectangle with water. Continue to roll over it and completely seal the cone.

7. Repeat with the remaining nori sheets and fillings. Serve.

Storage: Wrap temaki rolls tightly in plastic wrap and store in the refrigerator for up to 2 days.

Potato Frankie Rolls 🔺

Makes 8 to 10 rolls ■ *Ready in 40 minutes*

Frankies are a popular street food in India. They are made from chapati, a flatbread, which are filled with potatoes that have been cooked in spices and pickled raw onions and rolled up. This oil-free version uses tortillas because it's nearly impossible to find oil-free Indian flatbreads. Ground New Mexico chile is a mild powder and gives a nice red color to the dish, but any mild ground chiles can be used instead. Indian black salt, or kala namak, *has a sulfuric smell that is reminiscent of eggs. It's used extensively in Indian and other Asian cuisines, mostly in the form of a garnish or in spice blends, sauces, and pickles.*

FOR THE QUICK CHILI SAUCE

1 cup canned diced tomatoes, with their juice

1 teaspoon garlic powder

1 teaspoon onion powder

1 teaspoon ground New Mexico chile, or to taste

A few dashes of hot sauce, or to taste (optional)

Sea salt

FOR THE ROLLS

1 small onion, cut into ½-inch dice (about 1 cup)

1 tablespoon fresh lemon juice (from ½ lemon)

4 medium Yukon Gold potatoes (about 2 pounds), scrubbed and cut into 1½-inch pieces

2 teaspoons grated fresh ginger

4 small garlic cloves, minced (about 2 teaspoons)

1 teaspoon garam masala

1. Prepare the chili sauce: In a blender, place the diced tomatoes, garlic powder, onion powder, ground chile, hot sauce (if using), and salt to taste. Blend until smooth.

2. Transfer the sauce to a small pan and cook over low heat until the color darkens and the flavors merge, 5 to 10 minutes. Remove from the heat and let cool. (The sauce can be made in advance and stored in an airtight container in the refrigerator for 4 to 5 days.)

3. Make the rolls: In a small bowl, place the onion and lemon juice and stir to coat completely. Set aside.

4. Place a steamer basket in a large pot and add about 2 inches of water to the pot. Cover and bring to a simmer. Place the potatoes in the steamer, cover, and steam until cooked and tender when pierced with a fork, about 20 minutes. Transfer the potatoes to a large

2 pinches of ground turmeric

2 pinches of Indian black salt (optional)

Sea salt and freshly ground black pepper

2 small celery stalks, finely chopped (about ½ cup)

2 scallions, white and green parts, thinly sliced (about ½ cup)

¼ cup finely chopped fresh cilantro

8 to 10 (10-inch) whole wheat tortillas

bowl and use a potato masher to mash them. Set aside.

5. In a large sauté pan, place the ginger, garlic, and ½ cup water and cook over medium heat until softened, about 5 minutes.

6. Add the garam masala, turmeric, black salt (if using), salt and pepper to taste, and the reserved potatoes. Mix well and cook until heated through and the flavors have blended, 5 to 10 minutes, adding water as necessary to keep the mixture from getting too thick.

7. Stir in the celery, scallions, and cilantro and remove from the heat.

8. Warm a tortilla for about 20 seconds on each side in a dry skillet set over medium heat. Or if you have a gas stove, place a tortilla straight over the flame for a few seconds on each side. Cover with a large damp cloth. Repeat with the remaining tortillas. Keep them covered until ready to use.

9. Place a tortilla on the work surface. Place a spoonful of the potato mixture in the middle, top with a spoonful of onion, and drizzle with the hot sauce. Roll up the tortilla. Wrap one end of roll in a piece of wax paper to make it easier to hold and to keep the stuffing in place. Repeat with the remaining tortillas, potatoes, onion, and hot sauce. Serve.

Storage: Wrap frankies tightly in wax paper and store in the refrigerator for up to 4 days.

Falafel Sandwiches 🛍 📷

Makes about 16 falafels (8 sandwiches) ■ *Ready in*
50 minutes (plus overnight for soaking the chickpeas)

Here is a case where using dried chickpeas is really the only way to go; canned chickpeas just don't yield the same crisp texture that soaked chickpeas do. Leave the bowl of soaking chickpeas in the fridge overnight so that there is no concern of the peas fermenting if left soaking for too long. These sandwiches are great as a packed lunch, with the sauce served on the side so it doesn't make the sandwich soggy. You can also serve the falafel patties over small slices of pita bread and drizzled with tahini sauce as appetizers.

FOR THE FILLING

1 cup dried chickpeas, rinsed
   and drained

1 small onion, roughly
   chopped (about 1 cup)

1 cup broccoli florets in 1-inch
   pieces (about 3 ounces)

1 cup fresh parsley leaves

10 small garlic cloves

¼ cup ground flaxseed

¼ cup whole wheat flour

4 teaspoons ground coriander

4 teaspoons ground cumin

2 teaspoons baking powder

2 teaspoons ground turmeric

2 tablespoons fresh lemon
   juice (from 1 lemon)

Sea salt and freshly ground
   black pepper

4 scallions, white and green
   parts, thinly sliced (about
   1 cup)

1. Make the filling: Place the rinsed chickpeas in a bowl and cover generously with cold water. Set in the refrigerator to soak overnight.

2. Preheat the oven to 350°F. Line a baking sheet with parchment paper.

3. Drain the chickpeas and transfer to a food processor. Add the onion, broccoli, parsley, garlic, ground flaxseed, flour, coriander, cumin, baking powder, turmeric, lemon juice, and salt and pepper to taste. Pulse to a coarse mixture.

4. Transfer to a large bowl. Add the scallions and mix well.

5. Scoop out a rounded ¼ cup of the mixture and form into a patty 2 inches wide and 1 inch thick. Place on the prepared baking sheet and continue with the remaining mixture to make 16 patties total.

6. Bake in the oven until the tops are crisp and brown, about 30 minutes.

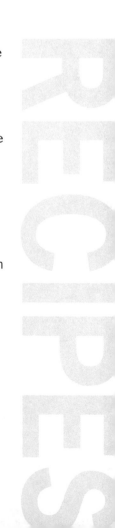

FOR SERVING
4 (6-inch) pita breads
2 medium tomatoes, thinly
sliced (about 2 cups)
2 cups shredded lettuce
1 cup Tahini Sauce
(page 241), or as needed

7. Flip the patties over and bake until the tops are browned, about 10 minutes more.

8. Assemble the pitas: Heat a griddle or skillet over medium heat and warm the pita breads on both sides. Cut each pita bread in half crosswise and open the pocket.

9. Stuff each pita with 1 or 2 slices of tomato and some lettuce. Place 2 falafels in each pocket and drizzle with the tahini sauce. Serve.

Storage: Wrap the sandwiches tightly in wax paper and store in the refrigerator for up to 2 days.

RECIPES

Spiced Sweet Potato Tacos 📷

Makes 12 to 16 tacos ■ Ready in 35 minutes

These are a favorite of my friend Judy Micklewright's six-year-old daughter,
Becky, who could not stop eating them the first time I served them to her.
Cutting the sweet potato into wedges makes them stay put in the tacos.

1 very large sweet potato
(about 1 pound)

½ small red onion, cut into
¼-inch dice (about ½ cup)

2 small garlic cloves, minced
(about 1 teaspoon)

1 (15-ounce) can pinto or
black beans, rinsed and
drained (about 1½ cups)

½ cup frozen sweet corn
kernels, rinsed

½ teaspoon ground cumin

½ teaspoon ground ancho
chile, or to taste

Sea salt

12 to 16 corn tortillas

1 ripe Hass avocado, pitted
and peeled

2 Roma (plum) tomatoes,
cored and cut into ¼-inch
dice (about 1 cup)

3 scallions, white and green
parts, thinly sliced (about
¾ cup)

¼ cup finely chopped fresh
cilantro

2 tablespoons fresh lime juice
(from 1 lime)

1. Cut the sweet potato lengthwise into
   ½- to ¾-inch-thick sticks.

2. Place a steamer basket in a sauté pan, and
   add 1 to 2 inches of water to the pan. Cover
   and bring to a simmer. Place the sweet potato
   wedges in the steamer, cover, and steam until
   the sweet potato is tender when pierced but
   not too soft, 7 to 10 minutes, making sure not
   to overcook. Remove the sweet potato from the
   pot and set aside.

3. In a large skillet, place the onion, garlic, and
   2 tablespoons water. Cover and cook over
   low heat until the onion is translucent, about
   10 minutes.

4. Add the reserved sweet potato, the beans, corn,
   cumin, ground chile, and salt to taste. Gently
   fold to coat the sweet potato with the spices.
   Cook over medium-low heat until heated
   through, 5 to 7 minutes. Remove from the heat.

5. Line a plate with a large, clean, damp dish
   towel. Warm the tortillas one at a time for about
   20 seconds on each side in a dry skillet set over

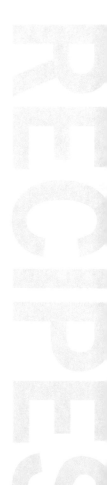

medium heat. Or if you have a gas stove, place a tortilla straight over the flame for a few seconds on each side. As you heat the tortillas, stack them on the damp towel and cover with the towel to retain moisture.

6. Place the avocado in a small bowl and use a fork to gently mash it.

7. Assemble the tacos: Spread some avocado on half of each tortilla. Spoon some beans and sweet potato on top, then add the tomatoes, scallions, and cilantro. Drizzle with some lime juice.

   Fold each tortilla in half over the filling. Serve at once.

Stacked Vegetable Sandwiches 🥪

Makes 10 sandwiches ▪ Ready in 50 minutes

These vegetable sandwiches are a popular street food in Mumbai, India, where they are cut into bite-size pieces and served wrapped in newspaper. The cilantro chutney gives them a unique savory flavor that is neither too spicy nor too intense, so even kids like it. These can be made ahead, ready for packed lunches or quick snacks.

2 large russet potatoes (about 1½ pounds), peeled and cut crosswise in half

2 medium beets (about 1 pound), peeled and cut crosswise in half

2 medium cucumbers (about 1 pound)

1 medium red onion (about ½ pound)

2 medium tomatoes (about ¾ pound)

1½ cups Cilantro Lime Chutney (page 239)

20 slices whole wheat bread

Sea salt and freshly ground black pepper

1. Place a steamer basket in a deep pan, such as a Dutch oven, and add 1 to 2 inches of water to the pan. Cover and bring to a simmer. Place the potatoes and beets in the steamer (don't let them touch each other if you want to keep the potatoes white). Cover and steam for 20 to 25 minutes, until they are tender when pierced, but not too soft. Set aside to cool completely.

2. Slice the tomatoes, cucumbers, and onion as thin as you can (ideally into rounds ⅛ to ¼ inch thick).

3. Spread half the chutney on one side of 10 bread slices. Layer the vegetables on top of each slice as follows: potatoes, beets, cucumbers, onion, and tomatoes. Sprinkle with salt and pepper to taste.

4. Spread the remaining chutney on one side of the remaining slices of bread and place them chutney side down on top of the tomatoes.

5. Cut each sandwich into 4 pieces. Serve.

Storage: Wrap the sandwiches tightly with wax paper and store in the refrigerator for up to 2 days.

Deviled Sandwiches 🥪

Makes 9 sandwiches (about 3 cups filling) ■ *Ready in 30 minutes*

*The filling for the Deviled Potatoes (page 183) is so good that it seems a shame
not to use it elsewhere, so we came up with these aptly named sandwiches.
They are excellent for packed lunches, and they're good enough to serve
a crowd at a party; simply cut each sandwich into smaller triangles.*

1 large Yukon Gold potato
(about ¾ pound), peeled and
cut into 1½-inch pieces

½ cup unsweetened,
unflavored plant milk or
water

¼ teaspoon prepared yellow
mustard

Pinch of ground turmeric

Pinch of black salt (optional)

1 (14-ounce) can hearts of
palm, drained and finely
chopped (about 1¼ cups)

1 small celery stalk, finely
chopped (about ¼ cup)

1 scallion, white and green
parts, thinly sliced (about
¼ cup)

Sea salt and freshly ground
white pepper

18 slices whole wheat bread

9 lettuce leaves, cleaned
(optional)

2 medium tomatoes, thinly
sliced (about 2 cups;
optional)

1. Place a steamer basket in a sauté or saucepan,
   and add 1 to 2 inches of water to the pan. Cover
   and bring to a simmer. Place the potato in the
   steamer, cover, and steam until very tender
   when pierced with a fork, 15 to 20 minutes.
   Remove from the heat and let cool.

2. Transfer the potato to a blender. Add the milk,
   mustard, turmeric, and black salt (if using).
   Pulse until smooth.

3. Transfer to a medium bowl. Stir in the hearts
   of palm, celery, scallion, and salt and pepper to
   taste.

4. Lay half the bread slices on a clean work
   surface. On each slice place a lettuce leaf and
   a couple of tomato slices (if using). Top each
   with ⅓ cup potato stuffing, then cover with the
   remaining bread slices.

5. If serving at once, slice in half and serve.

Storage: Wrap the sandwiches tightly in wax paper and store in
the refrigerator for up to 2 days.

SALADS

Beet, Fennel, and Red Rice Salad with Toasted Pumpkin Seeds

Makes about 6 cups ■ *Ready in 45 minutes*

Use Bhutanese red rice here for its especially soft texture and nutty flavor. It also has the advantage of cooking faster than brown rice, which certainly adds to its appeal. Buying precooked beets and roasted pumpkins can further simplify this already simple recipe. Serve this salad warm or cold as a side dish. Top it with some cooked beans to make a hearty one-dish meal.

¼ cup unsalted pumpkin seeds

1 cup dry red rice, washed and rinsed

1 small beet, peeled and cut into ¼-inch dice (about 1 cup)

2 small shallots, finely chopped (about ⅓ cup)

½ cup finely chopped fresh cilantro

3 tablespoons fresh lemon juice (from 1½ lemons)

1½ tablespoons white wine vinegar

½ tablespoon finely grated fresh ginger

½ small fennel bulb, very thinly sliced lengthwise (about 1 cup)

Sea salt and freshly ground black pepper

1. Preheat the oven to 250°F. Line a baking sheet with parchment paper.

2. Place the pumpkin seeds on the prepared baking sheet and toast for 15 to 20 minutes, or until lightly browned, shaking the baking sheet to move the seeds around midway through cooking. Transfer the seeds to a plate to cool.

3. Meanwhile, in a medium saucepan, bring the rice and 1½ cups water to a boil over medium heat. Reduce the heat, cover the pan, and simmer for 20 minutes. Remove the pan from the heat and let stand, covered, for 10 minutes.

4. Place a steamer basket in a sauté or saucepan and add 1 to 2 inches of water to the pan. Cover and bring to a simmer. Place the beet in the steamer, cover, and steam until tender when

pierced with a sharp knife, 10 to 15 minutes. Set the beet aside.

5. Place the shallots, cilantro, lemon juice, vinegar, and ginger in a large bowl and mix well. Add the warm rice, reserved beet, pumpkin seeds, and fennel, and salt and pepper to taste and mix well until combined. Serve warm or at room temperature. Or, to serve chilled, refrigerate until cold.

Storage: Store in an airtight container in the refrigerator for up to 2 days.

RECIPES

FORKS OVER KNIVES FAMILY

RECIPES

Quinoa Salad with Herbed Croutons 🛍

Makes about 10 cups ■ Ready in 30 minutes

This salad is a good make-ahead dish. It's actually best prepared at least an hour ahead of time and stored in the refrigerator before serving. This gives the vegetables a chance to meld and release more of their juices, which become a light dressing. The baked croutons add extra crunch and zesty flavor here; they are also good as a garnish for soups and for stuffing peppers or squash.

FOR THE CROUTONS
4 slices whole-grain bread, frozen
1 tablespoon nutritional yeast
1 teaspoon Italian seasoning
Sea salt and freshly ground black pepper

FOR THE SALAD
½ small red onion, finely chopped (about ½ cup)
2 Roma (plum) tomatoes, cut into ¼-inch dice (about 1 cup)
1 small cucumber, cut into ¼-inch dice (about ¾ cup)
1 to 2 tablespoons chopped fresh parsley
2 tablespoons fresh lemon juice (from 1 lemon)
1 cup broccoli florets in ½-inch pieces (about 3 ounces)
4 cups cooked quinoa (from about 1⅓ cups dry quinoa)
1 small head romaine lettuce, shredded (about 4 cups)
Sea salt and freshly ground black pepper

1. Preheat the oven to 350°F. Line a baking sheet with parchment paper.

2. Make the croutons: Use a sharp knife to cut the frozen bread into ½- to ¾-inch dice. Transfer to a medium bowl. Sprinkle the nutritional yeast, Italian seasoning, and salt and pepper to taste evenly over the bread. Toss gently to mix. (The moisture in the frozen bread will allow the seasoning to stick to it; if not using frozen bread, spray the cubes lightly with water before adding the seasonings.)

3. Spread the bread cubes evenly on the prepared baking sheet. Bake until crisp and slightly brown, 15 to 20 minutes. Let cool completely.

4. Make the salad: In a large salad bowl, place the onion, tomatoes, cucumber, parsley, and lemon juice. Toss gently to combine. Let stand in the refrigerator for 20 minutes.

5. Meanwhile, bring ½ cup water to a boil over medium heat in a small saucepan. Add the broccoli, cover the pan, and cook until slightly

softened, 5 to 7 minutes. Drain and let cool (or run under cold water for faster cooling).

6. Add the broccoli, croutons, quinoa, and romaine lettuce to the salad bowl. Mix well. Season to taste with salt and pepper.

7. Serve at once or chill in the refrigerator for at least 60 minutes and up to overnight before serving.

Storage: Store the croutons in an airtight container at room temperature for up to 10 days. Store leftover salad in an airtight container in the refrigerator for up to 1 day.

RECIPES

RECIPES

Israeli Couscous and Kale Salad 📷

Makes about 6 cups ■ *Ready in 40 minutes*

I really like how easy it is to cook Israeli couscous, and I love the way it absorbs and carries the flavors of the spices. Kids go for these little balls of pasta. Add some cooked chickpeas to make it a heartier meal.

½ bunch kale, thick stems removed, leaves chopped fine (about 2 cups)

3 tablespoons fresh lime juice (from 1½ limes)

1 cup Vegetable Stock (page 262) or no-oil, low-sodium store-bought

½ small onion, finely chopped (about ½ cup)

2 small garlic cloves, minced (about 1 teaspoon)

½ teaspoon curry powder

¼ teaspoon ground cumin

¼ teaspoon sweet or mild paprika

1 cup whole wheat Israeli couscous

½ medium tomato, cored and cut into ¼-inch pieces (about ½ cup)

½ red or orange bell pepper, cored, seeded, and cut into ¼-inch pieces (about ½ cup)

¼ medium cucumber, cut into ¼-inch pieces (about ½ cup)

4 scallions, white and green parts, thinly sliced (about 1 cup)

¼ cup finely chopped fresh parsley

1. In a medium bowl, place the kale and lime juice. Mix well so the leaves are well coated. Set aside.

2. In a large saucepan, place the stock, onion, garlic, curry powder, cumin, and paprika. Bring to a boil over medium heat and add the couscous. Cook over medium heat, uncovered, until the liquid has been absorbed and the couscous is al dente, 5 to 10 minutes. Add 1 to 2 tablespoons water toward the end of cooking if the liquid is absorbed and the couscous starts to stick to the pan. Transfer to a large bowl and let cool.

3. Add the reserved kale to the bowl with the couscous along with the tomato, bell pepper, cucumber, scallions, parsley, basil, raisins, pine nuts, and salt and pepper to taste. Mix well and adjust the seasoning. Chill in the refrigerator until ready to serve.

Storage: Store in an airtight container in the refrigerator for up to 3 days.

3 tablespoons finely chopped fresh basil

2 tablespoons raisins or currants

2 tablespoons pine nuts, toasted (see right)

Sea salt and freshly ground black pepper

Toasting Nuts

Toasting deepens the flavor of nuts and adds a nice roasty taste to whatever dishes they're used in.

To toast a small amount of nuts, place them in a medium skillet and toast over medium-low heat, stirring frequently, until lightly browned and fragrant, 4 to 7 minutes.

For large batches, spread the nuts on a baking sheet and toast in a 250°F oven for 15 to 20 minutes, stirring occasionally. Watch the nuts carefully so that they don't burn. Immediately transfer them to a plate to stop the cooking and let stand until cool.

Asian Rainbow Salad

Makes about 4 cups ■ *Ready in 30 minutes*

Seaweed is a staple of many Asian cuisines, and for good reason. Its crisp-tender texture is appealing and its flavor is bright. But there's not just one kind of seaweed, there are hundreds—although only a fraction of those are commonly used in the United States. This salad uses dried hijiki, which can be found in Japanese and Korean markets. This is a relatively quick salad to make, but the hijiki requires a few minutes to soak. If you don't have time for that step, sprinkle some toasted nori flakes on top of the salad instead, just before serving.

¼ cup hijiki (optional)

½ bunch kale or other hearty leafy green, shredded (about 2 cups)

1 cup shredded red cabbage (about ⅛ small cabbage)

1 yellow bell pepper, cored, seeded, and cut into ½-inch dice (about 1 cup)

2 medium carrots, cut into ½-inch dice (about 1 cup)

1 cup frozen shelled edamame

2 tablespoons low-sodium tamari or soy sauce

1 tablespoon Date Paste (page 265)

1 teaspoon grated fresh ginger

2 small garlic cloves, minced (about 1 teaspoon)

2 scallions, white and green parts, thinly sliced (about ½ cup)

1 tablespoon finely chopped fresh cilantro

1. If using the hijiki, place it in a small saucepan with 1 cup water. Soak for 20 minutes. Drain and return to the saucepan. Add 2 cups water and bring to a boil over medium-high heat. Boil for 5 minutes. Drain and set aside.

2. Place a steamer basket in a sauté or saucepan, and add 1 to 2 inches of water to the pan. Cover and bring to a simmer. Place the kale, cabbage, bell pepper, carrots, and edamame in the steamer. Cover and steam for 5 minutes, just until the vegetables wilt slightly. Remove from the heat and set aside for about 5 minutes to cool slightly.

3. In a large salad bowl, place the tamari, date paste, ginger, and garlic and whisk until well blended. Add the steamed vegetables, scallions, cilantro, and hijiki (if using). Toss well to combine. Serve at room temperature or chilled.

Storage: Store in an airtight container in the refrigerator for up to 3 days.

Spinach and Kidney Bean Salad

Makes about 6 cups ■ Ready in 15 minutes

This salad makes a great potluck dish because the vegetables stay fresh and crisp even when it is made in advance and stored in the refrigerator until ready to serve. If you have some leftover rice or another cooked grain, toss it in to turn this into a big, hearty meal.

1 (15-ounce) can red kidney beans, rinsed and drained (about 1½ cups)

1 large carrot, grated (about ¾ cup)

1 small cucumber, cut into ½-inch dice (about ¾ cup)

½ red bell pepper, cut into ½-inch dice (about ½ cup)

1 bunch fresh spinach, finely chopped (2 to 3 cups)

¼ cup finely chopped fresh parsley

½ to 1 cup Tahini Sauce (page 241)

Sea salt and freshly ground black pepper

1. In a large salad bowl, place the beans, carrot, cucumber, bell pepper, spinach, and parsley. (If not serving immediately, cover the bowl and store in the refrigerator until ready to serve.)

2. When ready to serve, pour the tahini sauce over the salad and toss until well coated. Season with salt and pepper to taste. Serve.

Storage/make ahead: The salad can be made ahead through step 1. Store in an airtight container in the refrigerator for up to 4 days.

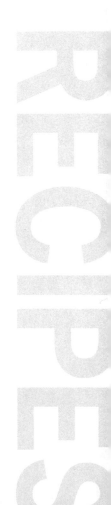

Chopped Vegetable Salad with Cheesy Dressing

Makes 7 to 8 cups ■ *Ready in 20 minutes (plus 1 hour for chilling)*

You might think this salad would be heavy because of the cheese-like dressing, but in fact it's surprisingly light and very tasty.

5 cups frozen mixed vegetables (about 24 ounces)

1¾ cups Cheesy Dressing (page 225)

2 scallions, white and green parts, thinly sliced (about ½ cup)

1 small head romaine lettuce, roughly cut (about 5 cups)

¼ cup finely chopped fresh cilantro

1. Bring a large pot of water to a boil. Add the vegetables, return to a boil, and cook until just tender, 5 to 7 minutes. Drain thoroughly and run cold water over the vegetables to cool them. Transfer the vegetables to a big bowl.

2. Add the dressing and scallions and toss to coat. Cover the bowl and place in the refrigerator for at least 1 hour.

3. When ready to serve, add the romaine lettuce and cilantro to the bowl and toss until the ingredients are well blended and the lettuce is well coated with dressing. Serve.

Storage: Store in an airtight container in the refrigerator for up to 3 days.

Glass Noodle Salad

Makes about 5 cups ■ *Ready in 20 minutes*

There are many varieties of fine noodles available, and any of them will work here. Glass noodles—also called cellophane noodles, Chinese vermicelli, or thread noodles—are made from the starch of mung beans or potatoes, among other things. You can also use rice vermicelli (thin noodles made from rice) or even angel hair pasta. You can find the noodles in well-stocked grocery stores or in Asian markets.

4 ounces dry glass noodles

⅓ cup frozen edamame

⅓ cup frozen corn kernels

⅓ cup frozen green peas

1 cup roughly chopped fresh spinach

1 to 2 tablespoons finely chopped fresh cilantro

½ Hass avocado, pitted, peeled, and cut into ½-inch dice

2 scallions, white and green parts, thinly sliced (about ½ cup)

2 tablespoons fresh lemon juice (from 1 lemon)

Grated zest of 1 lemon (about 1 tablespoon)

1 tablespoon low-sodium tamari or soy sauce

Sea salt and freshly ground black pepper

1. Bring a large saucepan of water to a boil over high heat. Cook the noodles according to package directions. About 1 to 2 minutes before the noodles are completely cooked, add the edamame, corn, and peas to the pan. Drain and rinse with cold water. If necessary, cut the noodles into roughly 2-inch lengths.

2. Transfer the noodles and vegetables to a salad bowl. Add the spinach, cilantro, avocado, and scallions.

3. In a small bowl, combine the lemon juice, lemon zest, tamari, and 2 tablespoons water. Mix well and pour over the noodles. Toss gently to coat all the ingredients in dressing. Taste and season to taste with salt and pepper. Serve at once or cover and refrigerate until chilled.

Storage: Store in an airtight container in the refrigerator for up to 2 days.

RECIPES

Red Cabbage Coleslaw

Makes about 8 cups ■ *Ready in 40 minutes*

Serve this coleslaw as a side salad, in a sandwich or a burger, or in a lettuce bowl. It will stay fresh stored in the refrigerator for 3 to 4 days, so it can become the week's condiment of choice, if you'd like. Use green cabbage instead of red for a more traditional look.

1 small red cabbage (about 1¾ pounds), cored and thinly sliced (about 12 cups)

4 tablespoons fresh lemon juice (from 2 lemons)

2 pinches of sea salt

½ cup frozen green peas, rinsed and drained

½ cup frozen yellow corn kernels, rinsed and drained

½ cup almond flour

2 tablespoons ground flaxseed

2 tablespoons Dijon mustard

2 tablespoons low-sodium tamari or soy sauce

2 to 3 tablespoons white wine vinegar

Dash of hot sauce (optional)

Pinch of freshly ground black pepper

2 medium carrots, grated (about 1 cup)

1 tablespoon finely chopped fresh cilantro

1. Place the red cabbage, 3 tablespoons of the lemon juice, and the salt in a large bowl. Use your hands to massage the lemon juice and salt into the cabbage. Let stand at room temperature for at least 30 minutes and up to 1 hour.

2. Meanwhile, in a small saucepan, bring 1 cup water to a boil over medium heat. Add the peas and corn, and cook until bright and just tender, about 2 minutes. Drain and rinse with cold water until cool. Drain thoroughly and set aside.

3. In a blender, place ¾ cup water along with the flour, ground flaxseed, mustard, tamari, vinegar, the remaining 1 tablespoon lemon juice, the hot sauce (if using), and the pepper. Blend until smooth; it may take a few minutes for the almond flour to be completely blended.

4. Pour the dressing into a jar with a tight-fitting lid and set aside.

RECIPES

5. Transfer the cabbage to a strainer and press with a ladle to squeeze out any excess liquid (or use your hands to squeeze it out).

6. Return the cabbage to the bowl. Add the carrots, the reserved peas and corn, and the dressing and mix well. Chill in the refrigerator until ready to serve. Stir in the cilantro just before serving.

Storage: Store in an airtight container in the refrigerator for up to 4 days.

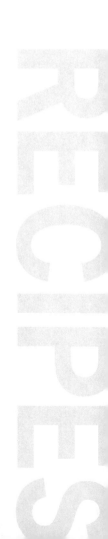

SIDE DISHES

Vegetable and Tofu Stir-Fry

Makes about 6 cups ■ *Ready in 30 minutes*

*Pressing the tofu to squeeze out the water it's been packed in
helps it absorb all the flavors of the other ingredients.*

1 (14-ounce) package firm tofu, drained

1 tablespoon grated fresh ginger

6 small garlic cloves, minced (about 1 tablespoon)

2 teaspoons ground coriander

1 teaspoon sweet or mild paprika

2 teaspoons grated lemon zest or 1 teaspoon dried lemon peel

Pinch of freshly ground black pepper (optional)

1 tablespoon no-salt-added tomato paste

6 scallions, white and green parts, thinly sliced (about 1½ cups)

1 (24-ounce) bag frozen stir-fry vegetables (about 5 cups)

Sea salt

2 tablespoons finely chopped fresh cilantro

2 tablespoons finely chopped fresh Thai basil

Steamed brown rice, for serving

1. Wrap the tofu in a clean white kitchen towel (sometimes the color of darker towels runs) or a paper towel. Place it in a colander set in a sink or on a plate. Fill a bowl that is slightly smaller than the colander with water and place it on top of the tofu to weigh it down. Let stand for 20 minutes. Cut the tofu into 1-inch cubes and set aside.

2. In a sauté pan, place the ginger, garlic, and ½ cup water. Cover and bring to a simmer over medium heat. Add the coriander, paprika, lemon zest, and the pepper (if using) and simmer for 2 minutes.

3. Meanwhile, in a small bowl, place the tomato paste and ¼ cup water and stir until blended. Add the tomato water, scallions, frozen vegetables, and salt to taste to the pan with the ginger and spices. Increase the heat to medium-high and cook the vegetables until softened, stirring frequently, 3 to 5 minutes, adding water

1 to 2 tablespoons at a time as needed to keep the vegetables from sticking.

4. Add the tofu to the pan and gently stir to coat. Cook until the tofu is heated through and has absorbed the spices, 5 to 7 minutes.

5. Transfer to a serving platter and garnish with the cilantro and Thai basil. Serve hot with brown rice.

Mashed Potatoes with Red Gravy

Makes about 6 cups mashed potatoes; about 4 cups gravy ▪ Ready in 35 minutes

*Mashed potatoes and gravy are the ultimate comfort food,
but they can take a little time to prepare. Using tomato
sauce as the base for the gravy gives it richness.*

FOR THE MASHED POTATOES

2½ pounds Yukon Gold
 potatoes (3 to 4 large),
 scrubbed and cut into
 1½-inch pieces

1 cup unsweetened,
 unflavored plant milk

1 tablespoon nutritional yeast

FOR THE RED GRAVY

1 small onion, finely chopped
 (about 1 cup)

1 small shallot, finely chopped
 (about 2 tablespoons)

8 small garlic cloves, minced
 (about 4 teaspoons)

2 cups Vegetable Stock
 (page 262) or no-oil,
 low-sodium store-bought
 or water

1 cup canned unsalted tomato
 sauce

2 ounces fresh mushrooms,
 trimmed and sliced (about
 1 cup)

1 tablespoon plus 1 teaspoon
 dried marjoram

⅛ teaspoon red pepper flakes
 (optional)

¼ cup oat flour

1 teaspoon nutritional yeast

Sea salt and freshly ground
 black pepper

1. Cook the potatoes: Place a steamer basket in a large pot and add about 2 inches of water. Cover and bring the water to a simmer. Place the potatoes in the steamer, cover, and steam until very tender, about 20 minutes. Remove the potatoes and the steamer basket from the pot, drain out all the water, and return the potatoes to the pot to keep warm until needed.

2. Meanwhile, make the gravy: In a large saucepan, add the onion, shallot, garlic, and ½ cup water. Cook, covered, over medium heat until the onion is translucent, about 10 minutes.

3. Stir in the stock, tomato sauce, mushrooms, marjoram, and the red pepper flakes (if using), and bring to a simmer. Simmer, uncovered, for 10 minutes.

4. In a small bowl, mix the oat flour and nutritional yeast with 1 cup water. Add the oat-flour slurry to the gravy and cook until the gravy has thickened to the desired texture, 5 to 10 minutes. Add salt and pepper to taste. Using a hand blender or a regular blender, blend the gravy until smooth.

5. Mash the potatoes: Transfer the warm potatoes to a bowl and mash them using a masher. In a small bowl, whisk together the milk and nutritional yeast. Add the milk to the mashed potatoes and stir well to blend.

6. Serve the mashed potatoes topped with a ladleful of gravy.

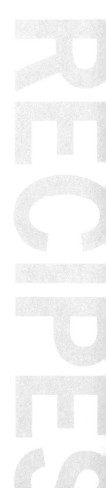

Savoy Cabbage with Mushrooms and Sesame Seeds

Makes about 4 cups ■ Ready in 30 minutes

This light sauté goes well with steamed grains or over noodles. The Savoy cabbage's tender leaves cook so much more quickly than regular green or red cabbage. You can certainly use the latter; if you do, just cook it a bit longer. Serve this cabbage in lettuce bowls for a fun presentation.

8 ounces shiitake mushrooms, tough stems trimmed, sliced (about 4 cups)

2 medium carrots, grated (about 1 cup)

2 scallions, white and green parts, thinly sliced diagonally into 1-inch-long strips (about ½ cup)

1 tablespoon grated fresh ginger

6 small garlic cloves, minced (about 1 tablespoon)

2 tablespoons low-sodium tamari or soy sauce

1 tablespoon arrowroot powder

Pinch of freshly ground black pepper

1 small Savoy cabbage (about 1¼ pounds), halved, cored, and thinly sliced crosswise (about 8 cups)

¼ cup chopped unsalted cashews

1 teaspoon sesame seeds

1 tablespoon finely chopped fresh cilantro

1. In a skillet, place the mushrooms, carrots, scallions, ginger, and garlic. Cook over medium heat, uncovered, until the mushrooms and carrots are soft and the liquid released from the mushrooms has evaporated, about 10 minutes.

2. Meanwhile, in a small bowl, prepare a slurry. Mix 2 tablespoons water with the tamari, arrowroot powder, and pepper.

3. Add the Savoy cabbage and the slurry to the skillet. Increase the heat to high and cook until the cabbage is tender, 5 to 7 minutes.

4. In another skillet, toast the cashews over medium heat until they are slightly brown (halfway toasted), 3 to 4 minutes. Add the sesame seeds and toast the seeds and nuts together until medium brown, 2 to 3 minutes more.

5. Transfer the cabbage to a serving bowl. Sprinkle the sesame seeds and cashews over the cabbage and garnish with the cilantro. Serve hot.

Roasted Stuffed Tomatoes 🛆

Makes 12 to 16 tomatoes; about 4 cups stuffing ■ *Ready in 50 minutes*

This is a good dish for a quick-to-table dinner or even a party, since the tomatoes can be stuffed in advance and baked just before serving. Drizzle with the cilantro chutney for a bright accompaniment or tahini sauce for a richer flavor.

1 small red onion, finely chopped (about 1 cup)

3 small garlic cloves, minced (about ½ tablespoon)

1 teaspoon dried thyme

1 cup cauliflower florets in 1-inch pieces (about 3 ounces)

1 cup broccoli florets in 1-inch pieces (about 3 ounces)

1 medium russet potato (about ½ pound), roughly chopped (about 2 cups)

½ cup frozen green peas, rinsed and drained

¼ cup finely chopped fresh basil

1 teaspoon sweet or mild paprika

2 cups cooked quinoa (from about ⅔ cup dry)

2 tablespoons pine nuts

1 tablespoon fresh lemon juice (from ½ lemon)

Sea salt and freshly ground black pepper

10 to 12 medium tomatoes (about 4 pounds)

Cilantro Lime Chutney (page 239) or Tahini Sauce (page 241), for serving

1. Preheat the oven to 400°F.

2. In a sauté pan, place the onion, garlic, thyme, and ¼ cup water. Cook over medium heat, covered, until the onion is cooked, about 10 minutes.

3. Meanwhile, in a food processor, pulse the cauliflower, broccoli, and potato until coarsely chopped. Add to the onion along with the peas, basil, and paprika. Cook until the flavors blend and the vegetables begin to soften, 5 to 7 minutes.

4. Transfer the mixture to a large bowl. Add the quinoa, pine nuts, lemon juice, and salt and pepper to taste. Mix well and adjust the seasoning.

5. Cut the top ¼ inch off the stem end of the tomatoes. Use a small spoon to scrape out the seeds and flesh from the tomatoes.

6. Fill each tomato with the quinoa and vegetable stuffing, dividing it equally among the tomatoes and placing the stuffed tomatoes in a large baking dish.

7. Bake until the tomatoes are cooked through and the stuffing is slightly browned on top, about 30 minutes. Serve hot with the chutney or sauce.

Storage: Store in an airtight container in the refrigerator for up to 3 days.

Chickpeazella Sticks 🛍 📷

Makes about 20 sticks ■ *Ready in 1 hour 40 minutes*

These might just remind you of mozzarella sticks! For best results, dry the squash, chickpeas, and rice in a hot oven as directed here. Too much moisture in these popular-with-kids sticks will prevent them from holding together when dipping.

8 ounces peeled and seeded butternut squash, cut into 1-inch pieces (about 1 cup)

1 cup cooked or rinsed and drained canned chickpeas

1 cup cooked brown rice (from about ¼ cup dry)

1 tablespoon finely chopped fresh parsley

½ tablespoon finely chopped fresh sage

¼ small onion, finely chopped (about ¼ cup)

1 small garlic clove, minced (about ½ teaspoon)

2 tablespoons nutritional yeast

1 tablespoon fresh lime juice (from ½ lime)

Sea salt and freshly ground black pepper

½ cup dry bread crumbs

Tomato Ketchup (page 237) or store-bought, for serving

1. Preheat the oven to 350°F. Line a baking sheet with parchment paper.

2. Place a steamer basket in a large pot, and add about 2 inches of water. Cover and bring the water to a simmer. Place the butternut squash in the steamer, cover, and steam until tender when pierced with a fork but not too soft, 5 to 7 minutes. Remove from the pot and spread on a baking sheet.

3. Spread the chickpeas and brown rice on the baking sheet with the squash. Place in the oven for 20 minutes. Remove from the oven, and let cool completely on the baking sheet, 15 to 20 minutes.

4. Transfer the chickpeas, rice, and butternut squash to a food processor. Add the parsley, sage, onion, garlic, nutritional yeast, lime juice, and salt and pepper to taste and pulse until the mixture is well blended and comes together into a slightly dry batter. (Alternatively, use a potato masher to mash everything together until well blended.)

5. Scoop out about 1 tablespoon of the mixture and use your hands to mold it into a 3-inch-long, ½-inch-thick rectangle. Roll the stick in the bread crumbs and place on the prepared baking sheet. Repeat with the remaining mixture and bread crumbs.

6. Bake until lightly browned, 30 to 40 minutes. Serve hot or warm with ketchup or your favorite dipping sauce.

Storage: Store in an airtight container in the refrigerator for up to 4 days or in the freezer for up to 1 month.

Red Lentil Fries 🔺

Makes about 4 dozen fries ■ Ready in 1½ hours

These fries started off as burgers and evolved into fries (you can certainly make them into burgers if you'd like!). They make good snacks or appetizers, and are great the day after in a packed lunch. Serve with any of the delicious dipping sauces listed here or with the sauce of your choice. Leftovers can be frozen.

1 cup dried red lentils, rinsed and drained

8 ounces button mushrooms, trimmed and cut into ¼-inch dice (about 3 cups)

1 medium sweet potato (about ½ pound), cut into ¼-inch dice (about 2 cups)

1 small onion, cut into ¼-inch dice (about 1 cup)

4 small garlic cloves, minced (about 2 teaspoons)

1 teaspoon grated fresh ginger

1 tablespoon ground coriander

¼ teaspoon ground cinnamon

⅛ teaspoon cayenne pepper

⅛ teaspoon freshly ground black pepper

1 cup finely chopped fresh cilantro

1 cup finely chopped fresh dill

1 cup finely chopped fresh spinach

2 tablespoons ground flaxseed

1 tablespoon low-sodium tamari or soy sauce

2 tablespoons fresh lemon juice (from 1 lemon)

1. In a large saucepan, place the lentils, mushrooms, sweet potato, onion, garlic, ginger, coriander, cinnamon, cayenne, and pepper. Add ½ cup water and bring to a boil over medium heat. Reduce the heat to low, cover the pan, and simmer for 30 minutes, or until the sweet potatoes and lentils are completely cooked and tender. Stir occasionally to prevent the mixture from sticking to the pan. Add water 1 to 2 tablespoons at a time only if necessary to prevent sticking.

2. Remove the pan from the heat. Using a masher, mash the mixture lightly; you want a coarse texture, so don't overmash.

3. Add the cilantro, dill, spinach, ground flaxseed, tamari, lemon juice, and salt and pepper to taste. Mix well and cook over low heat for 10 to 15 minutes, or until all the moisture has evaporated from the pan. Spread the mixture on a baking sheet and set aside to cool completely.

4. Preheat the oven to 400°F. Line two baking sheets with parchment paper.

Sea salt and freshly ground black pepper

Cheesy Dressing (page 225), Barbecue Sauce (page 238) or store-bought, or Tomato Ketchup (page 237) or store-bought, for serving

5. Scoop up 1 tablespoon of the cooled mixture and roll it into a stick about ½ inch thick and 3 inches long. Place the stick on a prepared baking sheet. Repeat with the remaining mixture.

6. Bake the fries for 20 minutes, or until they are crispy and brown on the underside. Flip the fries and bake for another 20 minutes, until firm and crispy all over. Serve hot with cheesy dressing, barbecue sauce, ketchup, or another dipping sauce.

Storage: Store in an airtight container in the refrigerator for up to 4 days or in the freezer for up to 1 month.

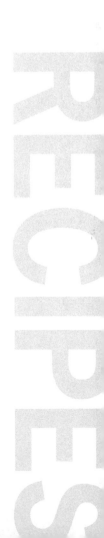

Crispy Potato Fries

Makes about 40 wedges ▪ Ready in 35 minutes

These fries taste good whether they're made with russet potatoes, sweet potatoes, or yucca. The sweet paprika and garlic powder add great color and zing, but you can skip them both if you prefer your crispy fries plain. On the other hand, to add a spicy kick, sprinkle them with ¼ teaspoon cayenne, or to taste.

4 large russet potatoes (about 3 pounds), scrubbed and each cut lengthwise into about 10 wedges

¼ cup fresh lemon juice (from 2 lemons)

2½ tablespoons sweet or mild paprika

2 teaspoons garlic powder

Sea salt and freshly ground black pepper

½ cup dry bread crumbs

Tomato Ketchup (page 237) or store-bought (optional)

1. Preheat the oven to 450°F. Line a large baking sheet with parchment paper.
2. Place a steamer basket in a large pot, and add about 2 inches of water. Cover and bring the water to a simmer. Place the potato wedges in the steamer, cover, and steam until the potatoes are tender when pierced with a fork but not too soft, 7 to 10 minutes, making sure not to overcook.
3. Meanwhile, in a large bowl, whisk together the lemon juice, paprika, garlic powder, and salt and pepper to taste. Add the hot potatoes and gently toss with the spice mix to coat evenly. Add the bread crumbs and quickly and gently mix with the potatoes.
4. Spread the potatoes on the prepared baking sheet. Bake in the oven for 10 minutes.
5. Remove the baking sheet from the oven and toss the fries. Return to the oven, and bake until the edges turn crispy and brown, about 10 minutes. Serve hot with ketchup or your favorite dipping sauce.

Storage: Store in an airtight container in the refrigerator for up to 4 days.

SOUPS AND STEWS

Minestrone

Makes about 15 cups ▪ Ready in 40 minutes

The first time I made this soup, I ate so much of it that I decided to double my recipe. This makes one great big pot of bean-and-pasta soup, and it is such a hearty meal that you will not need to cook anything else for dinner.

2 (15-ounce) cans kidney beans, rinsed and drained (about 3 cups)

1 medium onion, cut into ¼-inch dice (about 2 cups)

4 large celery stalks, cut into ½-inch pieces (about 2 cups)

8 small garlic cloves, minced (about 4 teaspoons)

2 teaspoons dried oregano

2 teaspoons dried basil

2 teaspoons dried thyme

2 teaspoons dried rosemary

20 ounces frozen mixed green beans and carrots (about 4 cups)

4 medium tomatoes (about 1½ pounds), cut into ½-inch dice (about 4 cups)

1 large zucchini, cut into ¼-inch-thick half-moons (about 2 cups)

1 (6-ounce) can no-salt-added tomato paste

Sea salt and freshly ground black pepper

3 cups (8 ounces) dry shell pasta

1. In a large stew pot, place the kidney beans, onion, celery, garlic, oregano, basil, thyme, rosemary, and 1 cup water. Bring the liquid to a boil over medium-high heat, then cover and cook over medium heat until the onion is translucent, 7 to 10 minutes.

2. Add the frozen green beans and carrots, tomatoes, zucchini, tomato paste, salt and pepper to taste, and 2 to 4 cups water to cover the vegetables. Bring to a boil over medium-high heat. Add the pasta and reduce the heat. Simmer until the pasta is al dente, 15 to 20 minutes, adding water if necessary to thin the soup. Serve hot.

Storage: If making this soup ahead, don't add the pasta. Cool the soup completely and transfer to an airtight container. Store in the refrigerator for up to 3 days or in the freezer for up to 1 month. When ready to serve, bring the soup to a simmer in a stew pot, stir in the dry pasta, and continue as directed.

RECIPES

Black Bean Chili 📷

Makes about 12 cups ■ Ready in 1¼ hours

The ingredient list here might look a little long, but please don't let that stop you from trying this delectable chili. There are only a few steps, and it is so chock full of vegetables, beans, and greens that all you need is some simple steamed grains or warm tortillas on the side to make this a very satisfying and filling meal.

5 medium tomatoes, cut into ½-inch dice or 3 (15-ounce) cans diced tomatoes, with their juice (about 5 cups)

2 red bell peppers, cored, seeded, and cut into ½-inch dice (about 2 cups)

½ medium red onion, finely chopped (about 1 cup)

4 small garlic cloves, roughly chopped (about 2 teaspoons)

4 teaspoons dried Mexican oregano

2 teaspoons ground cumin

2 (15-ounce) cans black beans, rinsed and drained (about 3 cups)

3 large celery stalks, cut into ¼-inch dice (about 1½ cups)

1 green bell pepper, cored, seeded, and finely chopped (about 1 cup)

1 cup fresh or frozen corn kernels

½ bunch kale, stemmed and roughly chopped (about 2 cups)

¼ cup finely chopped fresh cilantro

1. In a large stew pot or Dutch oven, place the tomatoes, red bell peppers, onion, garlic, oregano, and cumin, and cook over medium heat, stirring occasionally, for 20 minutes (the juices from the onion and tomatoes will be enough to keep the sauce from burning).

2. Remove from the heat and let cool for 10 to 15 minutes. In a blender in batches or using a hand blender, blend the sauce until smooth. Return to the pot.

3. Add the black beans, celery, green bell pepper, corn, kale, cilantro, lemon juice, paprika, chili powder, salt to taste, and 2 cups water to the pot. Bring to a boil over high heat. Reduce the heat to low and simmer until the greens are tender and the chili thickens, 10 to 15 minutes.

2 tablespoons fresh lemon
   juice (from 1 lemon)

2 teaspoons smoked paprika

¼ teaspoon chili powder,
   or to taste

Sea salt

Steamed grains or warm
   tortillas, for serving

4. Serve hot over steamed grains or with warm
   tortillas.

Storage: Cool the soup completely and transfer to an airtight
container. Store in the refrigerator for 4 to 5 days or in the
freezer for up to 1 month.

RECIPES

Roasted Carrot and Tomato Soup

Makes about 12 cups ▪ *Ready in 1¾ hours*

Roasting the vegetables gives this soup its deep, rich flavor. The simplicity of the flavoring and few steps compensate for the hour of roasting required. It's good just as is, but it is extra filling and tasty when ladled over gnocchi—or, if you want to keep it really simple, top each serving with a few herbed croutons.

4 medium carrots, cut into 1-inch pieces (about 4 cups)

8 to 10 Roma (plum) tomatoes (about 2½ pounds), quartered lengthwise

2 medium onions (about 1 pound), quartered lengthwise

2 small russet potatoes (about ½ pound), scrubbed and cut into quarters

4 to 6 small garlic cloves

2 tablespoons finely chopped fresh sage

2 tablespoons finely chopped fresh basil

2 teaspoons white wine vinegar

Sea salt and freshly ground white pepper

Gnocchi Dokey (page 192; no sauce) or oil-free croutons (optional)

1. Preheat the oven to 400°F. Line two baking sheets with parchment paper.

2. Spread the carrots, tomatoes, onion, potatoes, and garlic on the prepared baking sheets.

3. Bake until the vegetables are soft and very lightly browned along the edges, 50 to 60 minutes.

4. Transfer the vegetables to a stew pot. Add 8 cups water and the sage and bring to a boil over medium-high heat. Reduce the heat, cover the pot, and simmer until the flavors are blended, 10 to 15 minutes. Let cool slightly.

5. Transfer the soup to a blender (in batches, if necessary) or use a hand blender to blend until smooth, adding up to 2 cups water if desired for a looser soup. Return the soup to the pot.

6. Add the basil, vinegar, and salt and white pepper to taste. Heat until hot over medium heat. Serve hot, ladled over gnocchi or topped with croutons.

Storage: Cool soup completely and transfer to an airtight container. Store in the refrigerator for 4 to 5 days or in the freezer for up to 6 weeks.

Corn Chowder

Makes about 10 cups ■ Ready in 50 minutes

*Corn chowder is universally appealing, especially among children,
because of its sweet taste and creamy texture. Here you will find
that creaminess without the heaviness of traditional recipes.*

1 small onion, cut into ¼-inch
dice (about 1 cup)

6 small garlic cloves, minced
(about 1 tablespoon)

6 to 7 cups Vegetable Stock
(page 262) or no-oil,
low-sodium store-bought

6 cups fresh or frozen corn
kernels (from 6 fresh cobs
or about 24 ounces frozen)

1 large russet potato (about
¾ pound), scrubbed
and cut into ¼-inch dice
(about 3 cups)

1 medium red bell pepper,
cored, seeded, and cut into
¼-inch dice (about 1 cup)

1 teaspoon finely chopped
fresh parsley

1 teaspoon finely chopped
fresh thyme

⅓ cup almond flour

Sea salt and freshly ground
black pepper

1. In a large stew pot or Dutch oven, place the
   onion, garlic, and 1½ cups of the vegetable
   stock. Cover the pot and bring to a boil over
   high heat. Reduce the heat to low and simmer,
   covered, until the onion is translucent, about
   10 minutes.

2. Add the corn, potato, and 4½ cups of the
   remaining stock. Bring to a boil over medium
   heat. Reduce the heat and simmer until the
   potato is soft, 10 to 15 minutes.

3. Transfer half of the mixture to a blender and
   blend until smooth. Return to the pot. Add
   up to 1 cup stock to adjust the consistency if
   necessary.

4. Add the bell pepper, parsley, and thyme. Bring to
   a simmer and cook for another 10 minutes, until
   the flavors have blended and the pepper is tender.

5. Meanwhile, place the flour and ⅓ cup water in
   the blender and blend until smooth. Stir the
   almond cream into the chowder. Add salt and
   pepper to taste. Serve hot.

Storage: Cool soup completely and transfer to an airtight
container. Store in the refrigerator for 4 to 5 days or in the
freezer for up to 1 month.

RECIPES

Harira (Moroccan Chickpea Soup)

Makes 14 to 16 cups ■ *Ready in 1¼ hours*

Harira is a traditional Moroccan soup made with chickpeas, lentils, and a lot of spices. It is served with steamed rice or sometimes pasta. The list of ingredients here might look long, but the spices are primarily common ones and the rest of the ingredients are fresh veggies and pantry staples. The results are well worth the little bit of extra measuring!

1 cup dried brown lentils, rinsed and drained

1 medium onion, very finely minced or pulsed in a food processor (about 1 cup)

1 large celery stalk, cut into ¼-inch pieces (about ½ cup)

4 small garlic cloves, minced (about 2 teaspoons)

1 tablespoon grated fresh ginger

2 tablespoons sweet or mild paprika

1 tablespoon ground fennel seed

1 teaspoon ground turmeric

1 teaspoon ground cinnamon

2 pinches of freshly ground black pepper

2 pinches of cayenne pepper

2 (15-ounce) cans unsalted tomato sauce (about 3 cups)

1 (15-ounce) can chickpeas, rinsed and drained (about 1½ cups)

1. Place the lentils and 1 cup warm water in a small bowl and soak for at least 20 minutes and up to 1 hour. Rinse and drain.

2. Transfer the drained lentils to a large stew pot. Add the onion, celery, garlic, ginger, and 2 cups water. Bring to a boil over medium heat. Reduce the heat and simmer, covered, until the lentils are almost cooked (they'll be tender but still have a lot of bite), about 20 minutes.

3. Add the paprika, fennel seed, turmeric, cinnamon, pepper, cayenne, tomato sauce, chickpeas, frozen vegetables, cilantro, parsley, and 5 cups water. Bring to a boil over medium-high heat, then reduce the heat and simmer, covered, until the lentils are completely cooked, about 10 minutes.

1 (24-ounce) bag frozen mixed vegetables, including green beans, bell peppers, broccoli, and cauliflower (about 5 cups)

¼ cup finely chopped fresh cilantro

¼ cup finely chopped fresh parsley

1 tablespoon fresh lemon juice (from ½ lemon)

Sea salt

Steamed brown rice or cooked pasta, for serving

4. Add the lemon juice and salt to taste. Serve hot over brown rice or pasta.

Storage: Cool the soup completely and transfer to an airtight container. Store in the refrigerator for 3 to 4 days or in the freezer for 3 to 4 weeks.

Macaroni and Split Pea Soup

Makes about 12 cups ■ Ready in 1¼ hours

Split peas can take about an hour to cook; soak them overnight to cut the cooking time in half. Or, if you don't want to watch over a pot at all, put all the ingredients in step 1 in a slow cooker and cook on low heat for 3 to 4 hours. Then stir in the cooked macaroni and seasonings, and dinner is served!

1 pound dried green split peas (about 2 cups), rinsed and drained

1 medium onion, cut into ½-inch dice (about 2 cups)

4 large celery stalks, cut into ½-inch dice (about 2 cups)

6 small garlic cloves, minced (about 1 tablespoon)

2 teaspoons dried thyme

2 teaspoons dried marjoram

1 teaspoon mild curry powder

½ teaspoon ground turmeric

½ teaspoon dried sage

1 (16-ounce) bag frozen mix of carrots and green beans (about 3 cups)

1 cup dry whole-grain macaroni

¼ cup fresh lemon juice (from 2 lemons)

2 teaspoons white wine vinegar

¼ cup finely chopped fresh parsley

Sea salt and freshly ground black pepper

1. In a large stew pot, place the split peas, onion, celery, garlic, thyme, marjoram, curry powder, turmeric, sage, and 8 cups water. Bring to a boil over medium-high heat. Reduce the heat, cover the pot, and simmer until the peas are about three-fourths cooked, about 40 minutes.

2. Add the frozen carrots and green beans, and simmer, uncovered, until the split peas are cooked completely (they will be soft to the bite), about 20 minutes.

3. Transfer half the soup to a blender and blend until smooth. Return the pureed soup to the pot.

4. Meanwhile, bring a pot of water to a boil over high heat and cook the macaroni according to the package directions. Drain.

5. Stir the cooked macaroni into the soup along with the lemon juice, vinegar, parsley, and salt and pepper to taste. Bring to a boil over medium-high heat. Serve hot.

Storage: If making this soup ahead, don't add the macaroni. Cool the soup completely and transfer to an airtight container. Store in the refrigerator for 3 to 4 days or the freezer for 3 to 4 weeks. When ready to serve, bring the soup to a simmer in a stew pot while you cook the macaroni in a separate pot; continue as directed.

Lentil and Vegetable Stew

Makes about 10 cups ■ *Ready in 1 hour*

This simple stew is extremely versatile. It can be served by itself, on a bed of grains, or with bread. It is the base for Lentil Shepherd's Pie (page 182). And it's adaptable; you can use your own favorites in place of the ones here (use about 10 cups total in place of the zucchini, carrots, and green beans) or stir in a few handfuls of greens toward the end of cooking. Pass a bottle of hot sauce at the table for those who want to spice it up. To cut the cooking time in half, soak the lentils overnight.

1 cup dried brown lentils

1 small onion, cut into ¼-inch dice (about 1 cup)

4 medium tomatoes, cut into ¼-inch dice (about 4 cups)

3 large zucchini, cut into half-moons (about 6 cups)

2 large carrots, sliced (about 2 cups)

¾ pound green beans, trimmed and cut into ½-inch pieces (about 2 cups)

1 tablespoon Italian seasoning

1 teaspoon ground turmeric (optional)

Juice from 2 lemons (about ¼ cup)

Sea salt and freshly ground black pepper

1. Place the lentils and onion in a stew pot with 4 cups water. Bring to a boil over medium-high heat. Reduce the heat, cover the pan, and simmer until the lentils are almost cooked, 20 to 30 minutes.

2. Add the tomatoes, zucchini, carrots, green beans, Italian seasoning, and turmeric (if using). Cover and cook over medium heat until the vegetables are tender, 10 to 15 minutes, adding 1 to 1½ cups water as needed so the stew doesn't get too dry.

3. Stir in the lemon juice and salt and pepper to taste. Serve hot.

Storage: Let the soup cool completely and transfer to an airtight container. Store in the refrigerator for 4 to 5 days or in the freezer for 4 to 6 weeks.

Thai Vegetable Soup 📷

Makes about 9 cups ■ Ready in 30 minutes

Tamarind paste adds tangy sweetness and Thai basil has a stronger, spicier flavor than sweet Italian basil. Both can be found in Asian stores. These ingredients are a little unusual, but they are worth seeking out because they add something that really can't be provided by more common ingredients.

10 scallions, white and green parts, thinly sliced (about 2½ cups)

10 ounces king oyster or any other variety of fresh mushrooms, thinly sliced (about 4 cups)

2 tablespoons grated fresh ginger

12 small garlic cloves, minced (about 2 tablespoons)

1 (32-ounce) bag frozen mixed vegetables including carrots, green beans, broccoli, and cauliflower (about 6½ cups)

2 (13.5-ounce) cans light coconut milk

1 tablespoon tamarind paste

2 tablespoons grated lemon zest (from 2 lemons) or 1 tablespoon dried lemon peel

Sea salt and freshly ground white pepper

2 tablespoons finely chopped fresh mint

2 tablespoons finely chopped fresh Thai basil

2 tablespoons finely chopped fresh cilantro

Steamed brown rice or boiled noodles, for serving

1. Place the scallions, mushrooms, ginger, garlic, and 1 cup water in a large stew pot. Bring to a simmer. Cover and cook over medium heat until softened, 5 to 7 minutes.

2. Add the frozen vegetables, cover, and cook until they are tender but still have some bite, about 5 minutes.

3. Stir in the coconut milk, tamarind paste, lemon zest, and salt and white pepper to taste. Add water if necessary to cover the vegetables. Bring the soup to a boil over medium-high heat.

4. Garnish with fresh mint, basil, and cilantro. Serve hot ladled over brown rice or noodles.

Storage: If you are making this ahead, don't add the fresh herbs. Let the soup cool completely and transfer to an airtight container. Store in the refrigerator for 3 to 4 days or in the freezer for 4 to 5 weeks. Before serving, reheat and garnish with the fresh herbs as directed.

White Bean Winter Cassoulet

Makes 12 to 15 cups ■ Ready in 45 minutes

Traditional cassoulet requires long, slow cooking. This quick version gives tons of flavor (and smells amazing) in a fraction of the time. Replace the acorn squash with sweet potatoes or Yukon Gold potatoes for a creamier texture.

3 leeks, white and light green parts only, finely chopped (about 3 cups)

6 small garlic cloves, minced (about 1 tablespoon)

1 medium acorn squash (about 2 pounds), seeded, peeled, and cut into ½-inch dice (about 6 cups)

3 (15-ounce) cans diced tomatoes (about 4½ cups)

3 (15-ounce) cans white beans, rinsed and drained (about 4½ cups)

1½ tablespoons herbes de Provence

Sea salt and freshly ground black pepper

Steamed grains or bread, for serving (optional)

1. Place the leeks, garlic, and 1 cup water in a stew pot. Cook over medium heat until the leeks and garlic start to wilt and soften, 5 to 7 minutes, adding water 1 tablespoon at a time as needed to keep the vegetables from sticking.

2. Add the squash, tomatoes, beans, herbes de Provence, and 6 cups water. Bring to a boil over medium-high heat. Reduce the heat, cover, and simmer until the flavors are blended and the squash is completely cooked, 15 to 20 minutes. Add salt and pepper to taste.

3. Serve hot, with cooked grains or bread if desired.

Storage: Let the soup cool completely and transfer to an airtight container. Store in the refrigerator for up to 4 days or in the freezer for up to 4 weeks.

RECIPES

Creole-Style Chickpea Stew

Makes about 12 cups ■ *Ready in 1 hour*

Here's a hearty stew with a lot of flavor. Make a bigger meal by serving it over a bed of steamed grains or greens (such as kale or chard).

2 medium onions (about 1 pound), quartered

2 medium shallots, halved

4 small garlic cloves, minced (about 2 teaspoons)

1 large Yukon Gold potato (about ¾ pound), scrubbed and cut into ½-inch dice (about 3 cups)

1 pound button or cremini mushrooms, trimmed and sliced (about 6 cups)

2 large celery stalks, finely chopped (about 1 cup)

3 tablespoons Mild Creole Seasoning (recipe follows) or store-bought

2 red bell peppers, cored, seeded, and cut into ½-inch dice (about 2 cups)

2 (15-ounce) cans chickpeas, rinsed and drained (about 3 cups)

2 cups frozen green peas

1 quart Vegetable Stock (page 262) or no-oil, low-sodium store-bought or water

½ cup chickpea or whole wheat flour

Sea salt and freshly ground black pepper

Steamed quinoa or brown rice, for serving

1. Place the onion, shallots, and garlic in a food processor. Pulse until finely chopped.

2. Transfer the onion mixture to a stew pot and add the potato, mushrooms, celery, and Creole seasoning. Cook over medium heat for 10 minutes.

3. Add the bell peppers, chickpeas, peas, and vegetable stock. Bring to a boil over high heat.

4. In a small bowl, mix the flour with 1 cup water to form a slurry. Stir the slurry into the stew. Reduce the heat to low and simmer for 30 minutes. Add salt and pepper to taste.

5. Serve hot with steamed quinoa or brown rice.

Storage: Let the soup cool completely and transfer to an airtight container. Store in the refrigerator for 4 to 5 days or in the freezer for 4 to 6 weeks.

Mild Creole Seasoning

Makes about ¼ cup

Most store-bought blends of Creole spices have a bit of heat that may not appeal to kids. This blend is big on the flavor but easy on the hot.

2 teaspoons dried thyme

2 teaspoons onion powder

2 teaspoons garlic powder

1 teaspoon ground fennel seed

1 teaspoon sweet or mild paprika

1 teaspoon dried oregano

1 teaspoon dried lemon peel

1 teaspoon ground New Mexico or other very mild chile, or to taste

Pinch of cayenne pepper

Pinch of black pepper

In a small mason jar with a tight-fitting lid, mix the thyme, onion powder, garlic powder, fennel seed, paprika, oregano, lemon peel, ground chile, cayenne, and black pepper.

Storage: If the ingredients are fresh, the mixture will keep in the covered jar for at least 4 to 6 months.

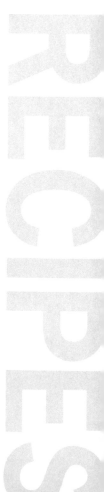

Summer Mint Cucumber Soup

Makes about 8 cups ■ *Ready in 15 minutes (plus chilling time)*

This began as a simple cucumber sauce, which tasted so good it deserved to be eaten with a spoon. The next step was obvious: find a way to transform this into a delicious soup. With some plant-based milk and vegetables, the transformation was complete!

1 medium-large cucumber (about 10 ounces), peeled if desired

2 (15-ounce) cans cannellini beans, rinsed and drained (about 3 cups)

¼ medium onion, cut into big pieces (about 2 ounces)

6 small garlic cloves

A ½-inch piece of jalapeño pepper, seeded (optional)

¼ cup fresh lemon juice (from 2 lemons)

2 cups fresh basil leaves

1½ cups unsweetened, unflavored plant milk

Sea salt and freshly ground black pepper

½ red bell pepper, cut into ¼-inch pieces (about ½ cup)

½ cup frozen yellow corn kernels, rinsed

2 tablespoons finely chopped fresh mint

1. Cut three quarters of the cucumber into 1-inch pieces (you should have about 1½ cups). Cut the remaining cucumber into ¼-inch dice (you should have about ½ cup) and set aside.

2. Transfer the 1-inch pieces of cucumber to a blender. Add the beans, onion, garlic, jalapeño (if using), and lemon juice. Blend until smooth.

3. Add the basil and blend again until finely chopped.

4. Add the milk and 1 cup water and blend just until mixed. Add salt and pepper to taste.

5. Transfer to a bowl or other container and stir in the reserved diced cucumber, the bell pepper, and corn.

6. Chill the soup until cold.

7. Taste for seasoning. Garnish with the mint and serve.

Storage: Store in an airtight container in the refrigerator for 3 to 4 days.

Baked Ziti 📷

Makes 1 (9 × 13-inch) casserole ■ *Ready in 50 minutes*

*I never knew about baked ziti (it's not a staple in India!) until my
boyfriend told me it was one of his favorite dishes when he was a kid.
A little tweaking to make his old favorite into a plant-based dish,
and now I can absolutely understand why he loved it so much!*

2 cups (8 ounces) dry ziti

½ medium cauliflower (about
1 pound), cored and cut into
¼-inch florets (about 4 cups)

1 large zucchini, thinly sliced
(about 2 cups)

3 cups Jimmy's Marinara
Sauce (page 235)

2 tablespoons finely chopped
fresh basil

2 cups Yukon Golden Cheese
(page 233)

1. Preheat the oven to 350°F.

2. Bring a large pot of water to a boil over high
heat and cook the ziti according to the package
directions. Five to 7 minutes before the end of
cooking, add the cauliflower and zucchini.

3. Drain well, then return the pasta and
vegetables to the pot. Add the marinara sauce
and half the basil. Stir to mix well.

4. Transfer the ziti to a 9 × 13-inch casserole dish
and smooth the top.

5. Spoon the cheese on top so that it almost but
not entirely covers the ziti. Bake for 30 minutes,
or until the cheese is lightly browned.

6. Garnish with the remaining basil. Serve hot.

Vegetable and Cheese Enchiladas

Makes 1 (9 × 13-inch) casserole ■ Ready in 1½ hours

Kids love these cheesy enchiladas. Don't feel obligated to use exactly the vegetables listed here; you can certainly substitute your kids' favorites. If you want to add some chopped greens such as chard or kale, the enchilada sauce and cheese will entice even picky eaters to give them a try.

FOR THE FILLING

1 small red onion, cut into ¼-inch dice (about 1 cup)

2 small garlic cloves, minced (about 1 teaspoon)

1 green bell pepper, cored, seeded, and cut into ¼-inch dice (about 1 cup)

1 medium carrot, thinly sliced (about ½ cup)

1 cup cauliflower florets in ¼-inch pieces (about 3 ounces)

1 cup frozen or fresh corn kernels, rinsed and drained

1 (15-ounce) can black beans, rinsed and drained (about 1½ cups)

½ teaspoon ground cumin

½ teaspoon dried Mexican oregano

1 tablespoon finely chopped fresh cilantro

1 tablespoon fresh lime juice (about ½ lime)

Sea salt

1. Preheat the oven to 350°F.

2. Make the filling: In a large sauté pan, place the onion, garlic, and ¼ cup water. Cover and cook over low heat, stirring occasionally, until the onion is translucent, about 10 minutes.

3. Stir in the bell pepper, carrot, cauliflower, corn, beans, cumin, oregano, cilantro, lime juice, and salt to taste. Cover and cook until the vegetables are tender, 10 to 15 minutes, adding water 1 to 2 tablespoons at a time as needed to keep the vegetables from sticking. Remove from the heat and set aside.

4. Make the sauce: In a blender, place the tomato paste, flour, chile powder, paprika, cumin, oregano, and garlic powder. Add 2½ cups water. Puree until blended and smooth. Transfer to a saucepan and bring to a simmer over medium heat. Reduce the heat to medium-low and cook until the sauce has thickened, about 10 minutes. Remove from the heat.

5. Add water if necessary to the cheese sauce so that it is pourable, and set aside about 1 cup of the sauce for finishing the dish.

**FOR THE QUICK
ENCHILADA SAUCE**

1 (6-ounce) can no-salt-added
   tomato paste

1 tablespoon oat flour

1 tablespoon ancho chile
   powder or to taste

1 tablespoon sweet or mild
   paprika

1 teaspoon ground cumin

1 teaspoon dried Mexican
   oregano

1 teaspoon garlic powder

FOR THE ENCHILADAS

Yukon Golden Cheese
   (page 233)

14 to 16 corn tortillas

2 scallions, white and green
   parts, thinly sliced (about
   ½ cup)

6. Assemble the dish: Spread half of the enchilada sauce on the bottom of a 9 × 13-inch casserole dish. Set aside the remaining sauce for finishing the dish.

7. Place one tortilla on a clean work surface. Spoon about ¼ cup sautéed vegetables and beans onto the tortilla. Spoon about 2 tablespoons of the cheese sauce on top. Roll the tortilla closed and place it folded side down in the casserole dish. Repeat with the remaining tortillas, sautéed vegetables, and cheese sauce.

8. Pour the reserved enchilada sauce over the enchiladas and top each one with a spoonful of the reserved cheese sauce. Sprinkle the scallions on top. Bake for 20 minutes. Serve hot.

Storage: You can assemble the enchiladas completely the day before and refrigerate for up to 1 day (just hold off on sprinkling the scallions on top). When ready to serve, sprinkle with the scallions and heat as directed. For longer storage, tightly wrap the casserole dish and freeze for up to 2 months. To thaw, place in the refrigerator for 1 day before serving. When ready to serve, sprinkle with the scallions, heat, and serve.

RECIPES

Baked Bean Casserole with Yams

Makes about 14 cups ■ Ready in 2½ to 3½ hours
(or 4½ to 6½ hours in a slow cooker)

These beans are a great leave-it-and-forget-it component of this dish, especially if you prepare them in a slow cooker—although the delectable smell emanating from the kitchen as they cook won't let you forget about them completely! They freeze beautifully, so you can make a double batch and freeze half for another meal.

4 (15-ounce) cans navy or cannellini beans, rinsed and drained (about 6 cups)

2 bunches Swiss chard, stems and leaves finely chopped (about 8 cups)

4 small shallots, finely chopped (about ⅔ cup)

2 cups Vegetable Stock (page 262) or no-oil, low-sodium store-bought

2 cups Tomato Ketchup (page 237) or store-bought

¼ cup no-salt-added tomato paste

¼ cup vegan Worcestershire sauce

4 teaspoons onion powder

4 teaspoons garlic powder

1 teaspoon hot sauce, or to taste (optional)

Sea salt and freshly ground black pepper

2 large yams (about 1½ pounds), scrubbed and sliced into ¼-inch-thick rounds (about 6 cups)

1 tablespoon finely chopped fresh parsley

1. Preheat the oven to 250°F.
2. In a Dutch oven or other oven-safe pot with a tight-fitting lid, stir together the beans, chard, shallots, vegetable stock, ketchup, tomato paste, Worcestershire sauce, onion powder, garlic powder, hot sauce (if using), and salt and pepper to taste. Cover the pot and bake until the sauce thickens and the beans have absorbed the flavor, 2 to 3 hours. (Alternatively, stir together the ingredients in a slow cooker and cook on low for 4 to 6 hours.)
3. Meanwhile, place a steamer basket in a sauté or saucepan, and add 1 to 2 inches of water to the pan. Cover and bring to a simmer. Add the yams to the steamer, cover, and steam until tender but not mushy when pierced with a fork, 5 to 7 minutes.
4. Layer the yam slices on top of the beans to cover the surface. Bake, uncovered, until the yams are slightly browned, about 20 minutes. (If using a slow cooker, layer as instructed, then cook on low for 30 minutes.)
5. Garnish with parsley. Serve hot.

Polenta and Lentil Loaf with Chipotle Barbecue Sauce 📷

Makes 2 loaves ▪ *Ready in 1½ hours*

Chipotle-laced barbecue sauce gives nice zest and spice to this flavorful loaf. The loaves travel well and can be served hot or at room temperature, which makes this recipe great for parties and potlucks.

1 cup dried brown lentils

2 small onions, finely chopped (about 2 cups)

12 small garlic cloves, minced (about 2 tablespoons)

2 cups dry polenta

2 red bell peppers, cored, seeded, and finely chopped (about 2 cups)

2 tablespoons fresh lemon juice (from 1 lemon)

Sea salt and freshly ground black pepper

½ cup fine cornmeal

2 cups Barbecue Sauce (made with chipotle, page 238) or oil-free store-bought

1. Preheat the oven to 375°F. Line two (8½ × 4½-inch or 9 × 5-inch) loaf pans with parchment paper.

2. Place the lentils, onion, garlic, and 6 cups water in a large saucepan. Cover and bring to a boil over medium heat.

3. Stir in the polenta, bell peppers, lemon juice, and salt and pepper to taste. Cook over low heat until all the water has been absorbed and the lentils and polenta are tender, about 20 minutes, stirring frequently to prevent sticking to the pan.

4. Stir in the cornmeal and divide the mixture between the two loaf pans, smoothing the tops.

5. Coat the top of the loaves with ½ cup of the barbecue sauce, dividing it equally. Bake until the sauce has dried a bit, 30 to 40 minutes.

6. Let the loaves cool slightly in the pan, then cut into slices. Serve, passing the remaining barbecue sauce on the side.

Storage: Wrap the baked loaves tightly and store in the refrigerator for up to 3 days or in the freezer for up to 2 weeks. To easily defrost just what you want, cut the loaves into ½-inch-thick slices and place parchment paper between each slice before wrapping and freezing.

Stuffed Potato Puffs 🎒 📷

Makes about 1 dozen puffs ■ *Ready in 1½ hours*

Kids and adults alike love these very-easy-to-make and fun-to-eat puffs, which are a great appetizer or side dish. They're especially good for parties.

2 pounds Yukon Gold potatoes (about 4 medium), scrubbed

6 ounces green beans, minced (about 1 cup)

1 large carrot, minced (about 1 cup)

3 tablespoons fresh lime juice (from 1½ limes)

1 teaspoon garlic powder

Sea salt and freshly ground black pepper

2 tablespoons finely chopped fresh parsley or cilantro

½ cup unsweetened, unflavored plant milk

½ cup dry bread crumbs

Jimmy's Marinara Sauce (page 235) or Tomato Ketchup (page 237) or store-bought, for serving

Hot sauce, for serving (optional)

1. Preheat the oven to 400°F. Line a baking sheet with parchment paper.

2. Poke the potatoes with a knife in four or five places and place them on the baking sheet. Bake the potatoes until very tender when pierced with a fork, 45 to 50 minutes. Leave the oven on and at 400°F.

3. Meanwhile, in a large skillet, cook the green beans and carrot over medium-high heat until the vegetables are soft and all the moisture has evaporated, 5 to 10 minutes. Add 1 tablespoon of the lime juice, the garlic powder, and salt and pepper to taste; continue to cook for a few more minutes, until the flavors are well blended. Remove the pan from the heat. Add the parsley and mix well. Transfer to a bowl and set aside.

4. When the potatoes are done, transfer them to a cooling rack until cool enough to handle. Peel off and discard the skins and place the flesh in a large bowl. Add the remaining 2 tablespoons lime juice, the milk, and salt and pepper to taste. Use a potato masher to mash until smooth and well blended.

5. Line another baking sheet with parchment paper. Prepare a work station to form the puffs. Have ready the mashed potatoes and the green-bean-and-carrot stuffing. Spread the bread crumbs on a plate for breading.

6. Scoop up ¼ cup mashed potatoes and use your hands to pat it into a roughly ¼-inch-thick patty. Place 1 tablespoon of the stuffing in the middle of the patty. Fold over the edges of the patty to meet in the middle and cover the stuffing. Seal the puff and press it into a round ball, making sure that there are no breaks in the potato.

7. Roll the puff in the bread crumbs, ensuring the entire surface is covered, and place it on the baking sheet. Continue with the remaining mashed potatoes, stuffing, and bread crumbs. (The puffs can be refrigerated or frozen at this point; see storage.)

8. Bake until lightly browned, 25 to 30 minutes. Serve hot with marinara sauce or ketchup, or your favorite dipping sauce, and hot sauce (if using).

Storage: The puffs can be made ahead through step 7 and frozen on the baking sheet until solid. Transfer to a re-sealable bag and store in the freezer for up to 1 month. When ready to bake, arrange the frozen puffs on a baking sheet and bake until browned; it may take a few extra minutes. Or you can bake the puffs and store them in an airtight container in the refrigerator for up to 3 days; reheat until hot in a hot oven before serving.

RECIPES

Polenta Tempeh Casserole

Makes about 11 cups ■ *Ready in 1½ hours*

Feel free to substitute your favorite vegetables (or anything else you need to clear out of the crisper drawer) for the veggies here, and you can certainly use cooked beans or lentils in place of the tempeh. The remaining tempeh can be marinated and pan-toasted as described on page 217. Note that if the spices used in this casserole are too strong for your little ones, you may use 1 tablespoon Italian seasoning in place of the paprika, cumin, cinnamon, and cloves. Serve this as an accompaniment to hearty stews and soups.

FOR THE TEMPEH

1 leek, white and light green parts only, cut into thin rings (about 1 cup)

4 small garlic cloves, minced (about 2 teaspoons)

1 (16-ounce) bag frozen mixed vegetables (about 4 cups)

1 medium potato (about ½ pound), cut into ½-inch dice (about 2 cups)

1 medium tomato, cored and cut into ¼-inch dice (about 1 cup)

4 ounces tempeh (half an 8-ounce package), crumbled (about 1 cup)

1 teaspoon sweet or mild paprika

1 teaspoon ground cumin

¼ teaspoon ground cinnamon

¼ teaspoon ground cloves

1. Preheat the oven to 350°F. Have ready a 10-inch square or other 3-quart baking dish.

2. Make the tempeh: In a sauté pan, place the leek, garlic, and 2 tablespoons water. Cook over medium-low heat until the leek is wilted, about 5 minutes.

3. Add the frozen vegetables, potato, tomato, tempeh, paprika, cumin, cinnamon, and cloves. Cover and cook over medium heat until the vegetables are tender and all the water is evaporated, stirring frequently, 15 to 20 minutes, adding water 1 tablespoon at a time as needed to keep the vegetables from sticking. If necessary, uncover the pan and cook for 1 or 2 minutes to cook off any remaining liquid. Set aside.

4. Make the polenta: Bring the stock to a boil over medium-high heat in a large saucepan. While whisking constantly, add the polenta to the boiling stock in a slow and steady

FOR THE POLENTA

6 cups Vegetable Stock (page 262) or no-oil, low-sodium store-bought

1½ cups polenta

Sea salt and freshly ground black pepper

stream. Break up any clumps. Add salt and pepper to taste. Simmer, stirring frequently, until the stock is absorbed and the polenta is cooked, 20 to 25 minutes. It should be a spreadable consistency; if it is too dry, add a few tablespoons water. Evenly spread half of the polenta in the baking dish.

5. Spread the vegetables evenly over the polenta. Pour the remaining polenta over the vegetables and smooth the top.

6. Bake until the surface is a bit dry and crisp, 20 to 25 minutes.

7. Let cool slightly. Cut into squares. Serve warm.

Chickpea and Spinach Pizzas

Makes 2 (9 × 13-inch) pizzas ▪ Ready in 1½ hours

Making your own pizza dough is easy and fun to do with the kids when you have a foolproof recipe like this one (or you can double the recipe for gluten-free Cornmeal Pizza Crust [page 266]; or, if you're pressed for time, use your favorite whole-grain crust instead). When it comes time to top the pizza, the colorful and very yummy combination of chickpea and spinach is a hit, but naturally you can improvise—it's pizza!

FOR THE CRUSTS

2 cups unbleached all-purpose flour, plus more as needed

2 cups lukewarm (105°F to 115°F) water

2 (¼-ounce) packages active dry yeast (4½ teaspoons)

2 tablespoons Date Paste (page 265) or pure maple syrup

2 cups whole wheat flour

¾ teaspoon sea salt

Cornmeal, for dusting the pans

FOR THE SAUCE

1 (15-ounce) can unsalted tomato sauce

¼ medium onion, cut into big pieces (about ½ cup)

5 to 6 small garlic cloves

1 tablespoon dried rosemary

1 tablespoon dried oregano

½ teaspoon dried tarragon

½ teaspoon dried chives (optional)

1 tablespoon finely chopped fresh basil

Sea salt and freshly ground black pepper

1. Make the pizza crusts: In a medium bowl, place 1 cup of the all-purpose flour, the lukewarm water, and the yeast. Stir gently just until combined. Whisk in the date paste. Cover the bowl with a clean kitchen towel and set in a warm place, such as by the stove or in a warm oven, until the mixture begins to froth, about 10 minutes. (If the mixture does not froth, it indicates that the yeast is not active; begin again with fresh yeast.)

2. In a food processor fitted with a dough blade, place the remaining 1 cup all-purpose flour, the whole wheat flour, the salt, and the yeast mixture. Pulse a few times and then blend into a cohesive dough, 60 to 90 seconds.

3. Transfer the dough to a large bowl. If it is very sticky, add all-purpose flour a little at a time and knead it in until the dough is not too sticky. Cover with a damp cloth and let rise for 20 minutes in a warm place.

4. Preheat the oven to 400°F. Line two baking sheets with parchment paper. Sprinkle a little cornmeal on the paper.

FOR THE TOPPINGS

1 (15-ounce) can chickpeas, rinsed and drained (about 1½ cups)

1 bunch fresh spinach, trimmed and coarsely chopped (about 4 cups)

4 ounces cremini or button mushrooms, trimmed and thinly sliced (about 1½ cups)

1 small zucchini, thinly sliced (about 1 cup)

2 tablespoons nutritional yeast

5. Sprinkle some all-purpose flour on a clean work surface. Transfer the dough to the floured surface and knead gently to let the air out. Divide the dough in half and set aside one half under a cloth. Use a rolling pin or your hands to roll or stretch the other half into a large 9 × 13-inch rectangle. Transfer to a prepared baking sheet and repeat with the other dough half. Cover the dough with a damp cloth and let rise for 10 minutes.

6. Use a fork to poke a few holes in the dough. Bake the crusts for 10 minutes. (You can refrigerate or freeze the crusts at this point; see Storage.)

7. Make the sauce: In a blender, place the tomato sauce, onion, garlic, rosemary, oregano, tarragon, chives (if using), basil, and salt and pepper to taste. Blend into a smooth sauce.

8. Assemble the pizzas: Remove the crusts from the oven and divide the tomato sauce evenly between them, spreading it out. Divide the chickpeas, spinach, mushrooms, and zucchini between them. Sprinkle each pizza with 1 tablespoon nutritional yeast.

9. Bake until the toppings are well cooked and the edges of the crust are browned, 25 to 30 minutes. Serve hot.

Storage: Bake the crusts through step 6. Let cool and wrap them tightly, placing parchment between them if you are wrapping them together. Refrigerate for 3 to 4 days or freeze for up to 1 month. Tightly wrap leftover pizza in wax paper and store in the refrigerator for up to 2 days. Reheat in a preheated 350°F oven for 20 minutes.

Lentil Shepherd's Pie

Makes 1 (9 × 13-inch) casserole ■ *Ready in 1 hour*

This shepherd's pie is a great dish to include in a week's planning because it's made from different components—stew and gravy—that can be prepared in double batches earlier in the week and then half can be set aside for this casserole.

2 pounds potatoes (about 4 medium), scrubbed and quartered

1 cup Vegetable Stock (page 262) or no-oil, low-sodium store-bought

½ cup unsweetened, unflavored plant milk

2 small garlic cloves, minced (about 1 teaspoon)

1 tablespoon nutritional yeast

Sea salt

1 pinch of freshly ground white pepper

6 cups Lentil and Vegetable Stew (page 160)

Cremini Mushroom Gravy (page 236)

1. Preheat the oven to 400°F. Have ready a 9 × 13-inch casserole dish with 2½-inch-high sides and a baking sheet.

2. Place a steamer basket in a large pot, and add about 2 inches of water to the pot. Cover and bring the water to a simmer. Place the potatoes in the steamer, cover, and steam until the potatoes are tender when pierced with a fork, 20 to 25 minutes.

3. Transfer the potatoes to a large bowl and mash well while still hot.

4. In a medium bowl, whisk together the vegetable stock, milk, garlic, nutritional yeast, salt to taste, and the pepper. Pour over the potatoes and mix well.

5. Drain off any excess liquid from the stew, then spread the stew in the casserole dish. Spoon 2 cups of the gravy over the stew. Cover with the mashed potatoes and smooth them out.

6. Place the casserole dish on the baking sheet and bake until heated through and lightly browned on top, 50 to 60 minutes. Let stand 10 minutes before serving.

7. Meanwhile, heat the remaining gravy. Serve hot, with the gravy.

Deviled Potatoes 🥟

Makes 24 deviled potatoes ■ Ready in 1 hour

These yummy deviled potatoes are great finger food for parties. Black salt or rock salt is a common ingredient in South Asian cooking, which gives an eggy flavor to the filling. You can find it in Asian markets, or just use regular sea salt.

14 very small Yukon Gold potatoes (about 2½ pounds), scrubbed and halved lengthwise

1 cup unsweetened, unflavored plant milk

½ teaspoon prepared yellow mustard

Pinch of ground turmeric

Pinch of black salt (optional)

Sea salt and freshly ground white pepper

1 (14-ounce) can hearts of palm, drained and coarsely chopped (about 1¼ cups)

2 scallions, white and green parts, thinly sliced (about ½ cup)

1 teaspoon sweet or mild paprika

1. Preheat the oven to 400°F. Line a baking tray with parchment paper.

2. Place the potatoes cut side down on the parchment paper. Bake for 30 to 40 minutes, until the potatoes are completely tender when pierced with a fork. Let cool enough to handle.

3. Peel off and discard the skins from four of the potato halves. Add the halves to a blender.

4. Cut a thin slice off the bottom of each of the remaining halves so that they can sit steady.

5. Scoop out the centers of the potato halves to create a well, leaving ¼-inch-thick shells. Add the scooped-out bits to the blender. Place the potato cups on a serving tray.

6. To the blender, add the milk, mustard, turmeric, black salt (if using), and salt and pepper to taste. Pulse until smooth. Transfer to a large bowl. Add the hearts of palm and scallions to the bowl and stir until well mixed. Taste and adjust the seasoning.

7. Spoon the stuffing into the potato cups.

8. Just before serving, sprinkle with the paprika.

Storage: Store in an airtight container in the refrigerator for up to 2 days.

PASTA AND NOODLES

Mac 'n Cheese

*Makes 10 to 12 cups ■ Ready in 30 minutes on
the stovetop or 45 minutes if baked*

*Mac 'n cheese is classic "kid food," but the challenge is finding a plant-based
version that both kids and adults can love. This one fits the bill. Better yet, it's
quick and easy to make, and you can do it either on the stovetop or in the oven.*

**5 cups dry macaroni
(24 ounces), or about
10 cups leftover cooked
pasta (see Note 1)**

**4 cups Cheesy Dressing
(page 225)**

**½ cup unsweetened,
unflavored plant milk,
if needed**

**½ cup Cashew Crumble
(page 234; see Note 2)**

To make on the stovetop

1. Cook the macaroni according to the package
   directions. Drain and return the noodles to
   the pot.
2. Add the dressing and mix well. The mixture
   should be creamy; if it is too dry, add the
   milk a couple tablespoons at a time until the
   desired consistency is reached. If the mixture
   is too moist, cook over low heat until the sauce
   reaches the desired consistency.
3. Transfer the macaroni to a serving bowl and
   sprinkle the cashew crumble over it just before
   serving. Serve hot.

To make in the oven

1. Preheat the oven to 350°F.
2. Cook the macaroni according to the package
   directions. Drain and return the noodles to
   the pot.

3. Add the dressing and mix well. If the mixture is too dry, add the milk a couple tablespoons at a time to achieve the desired consistency.

4. Transfer the pasta to a 10-inch square or other 3-quart baking dish. Sprinkle the cashew crumble over the pasta. Bake until the crumble turns light brown, 15 to 20 minutes. Serve hot.

Note 1: To use leftover pasta, place it in the baking dish and add a little plant milk or water, stirring to loosen it. Bake for 20 minutes at 350°F. Alternatively, place the pasta and a little milk in a saucepan, stir, and reheat on the stovetop.

Note 2: To use bread crumbs instead of the cashew crumble, place ½ cup coarse dry bread crumbs and 1½ tablespoons mild white miso in a skillet and stir until they form a crumble. Lightly toast over low heat until the crumble is light brown, 2 to 3 minutes. Then crumble over the pasta as directed.

Spaghetti Marinara with Lentil Balls 📷

*Makes 20 to 22 lentil balls; about 8 cups
cooked pasta with sauce* ■ *Ready in 1¾ hours*

*These lentil balls take a little time to make, but they are well worth the
investment. In fact, they are a perfect weekend project for a memorable
Sunday dinner. Or you can make them in advance; they freeze beautifully.*

1 cup dried brown lentils,
rinsed and drained

3 small garlic cloves, minced
(about ½ tablespoon)

1 small onion, cut into ¼-inch
dice (about 1 cup)

8 ounces button or cremini
mushrooms, trimmed and
cut into ¼-inch dice (about
3 cups)

3 tablespoons low-sodium
tamari or soy sauce

2 tablespoons no-salt-added
tomato paste

1 tablespoon nutritional yeast

1 teaspoon dried oregano

1 teaspoon onion powder

¼ cup whole wheat flour

Sea salt and freshly ground
black pepper

1 pound dry whole-grain
spaghetti

Jimmy's Marinara Sauce
(page 235)

2 tablespoons finely chopped
fresh basil

1. Place the lentils and 1 cup water in a large
saucepan and bring to a boil over high heat.
Cover, reduce the heat, and simmer until
halfway cooked (beginning to soften but still
firm), about 15 minutes.

2. Uncover the pan and add the garlic, onion, and
mushrooms. Cover and cook until the lentils
are tender, about 15 minutes more. Uncover
and cook off any remaining liquid.

3. Stir in the tamari, tomato paste, nutritional
yeast, oregano, onion powder, flour, and salt
and pepper to taste and mix well. Cook over
low heat, uncovered, stirring frequently, until
all the water is absorbed and the pan is very
dry, about 10 minutes. (If necessary, place a
skillet or a flame diffuser under the pan to
prevent the lentils from scorching.)

4. Remove from the heat, spread the mixture on a
rimmed baking sheet, and let cool completely.

5. Preheat the oven to 250°F. Line a baking sheet
with parchment paper.

6. Scoop out 2 tablespoons of the lentil mixture
and roll into a ball. Place on the prepared

baking sheet and repeat with the remaining lentil mixture.

7. Bake the lentil balls until the outsides are slightly brown and crisp, about 45 minutes. (They can be frozen at this point; see Storage.)

8. Meanwhile, cook the spaghetti according to the package directions.

9. While the spaghetti is cooking, heat the marinara sauce in a saucepan over medium-low heat.

10. Drain the spaghetti and transfer it to a large bowl. Pour about 3 cups hot marinara sauce over the spaghetti, reserving the remainder to pour over the lentil balls.

11. Transfer the pasta to a large platter or individual plates. Place the lentil balls on top and spoon over the reserved marinara sauce. Garnish with the fresh basil. Serve hot.

Storage: The lentil balls can be made through step 7. Let cool completely, then transfer to an airtight container and freeze for up to 1 month. When ready to serve, preheat the oven to 350°F and bake the frozen lentil balls for 20 to 30 minutes.

RECIPES

Pasta alla Norma

Makes about 10 cups ■ *Ready in 40 minutes*

This Sicilian dish of pasta tossed with pan-fried eggplant and tomato sauce is much lighter when it is prepared without any oil or heavy cheese. You can replace the eggplant with an equal weight of zucchini, if you prefer.

2 medium eggplants (about 1½ pounds), cut into ¼-inch-thick slices

¼ cup dry bread crumbs

¼ cup almond flour

2 tablespoons nutritional yeast

2 tablespoons dried Italian seasoning

4 cups (¾ pound) dry short whole-grain pasta, such as penne or fusilli

3 cups Jimmy's Marinara Sauce (page 235)

2 teaspoons drained capers (optional)

2 teaspoons pitted sliced black olives (optional)

1 tablespoon finely chopped fresh basil

Sea salt and freshly ground black pepper

1. Preheat the oven to 375°F. Line two baking sheets with parchment paper.

2. Arrange the eggplant slices in a single layer on the baking sheets. Bake for 10 minutes.

3. Meanwhile, in a small bowl, stir together the bread crumbs, almond flour, nutritional yeast, and Italian seasoning.

4. Remove the eggplant slices from the oven, brush them with water, and pat the bread-crumb mixture on top. Bake until the topping is slightly brown and crisp to the touch, about 20 minutes more.

5. Meanwhile, bring a large pot of water to a boil over high heat. Cook the pasta according to the package directions.

6. Heat the marinara sauce in a large sauté pan over medium-low heat. Drain the pasta and add it to the marinara sauce. Toss to coat.

7. Place the eggplant on a large platter or individual plates and top with the pasta and marinara. Sprinkle on the capers and olives (if using), and scatter the basil on top. Season with salt and pepper to taste. Serve hot.

Note: To prepare this as a casserole, layer the eggplant slices on the bottom of a baking dish and top with the pasta and marinara sauce; bake at 350°F just until heated through.

Pasta Alfredo with Green Peas and Acorn Squash

Makes about 6 cups ■ Ready in 25 minutes

Any pasta works really well here. If your crew doesn't care for acorn squash, replace it with about 2 cups of another squash or starchy vegetable.

1 small acorn squash (about 1½ pounds), seeded, peeled, and cut into ½-inch dice (about 4 cups)

1 cup fresh or frozen green peas

2 cups Almond Milk (page 264) or unsweetened, unflavored store-bought, or as needed

1 (15-ounce) can cannellini or other white beans, rinsed and drained (about 1½ cups)

¼ cup nutritional yeast

2 small garlic cloves

½ tablespoon mild white miso

1 tablespoon fresh lime juice (from 1 lime)

½ teaspoon dried oregano

Sea salt and freshly ground black pepper

8 ounces dry pasta

1 tablespoon finely chopped fresh parsley

1. Place a steamer basket in a sauté pan, and add 1 to 2 inches of water to the pan. Cover and bring to a simmer. Place the squash in the steamer, cover, and steam until tender when pierced with a fork, 5 to 7 minutes. Transfer the squash to a large bowl and set aside.

2. Place the peas in the steamer, cover, and steam for 3 to 5 minutes. Add the peas to the squash and set aside. Remove the steamer basket and rinse out the sauté pan.

3. In a blender, blend 1 cup of the almond milk, the beans, nutritional yeast, garlic, and miso until smooth. Pour the sauce into the clean sauté pan, and add the lime juice, oregano, and salt and pepper to taste. Bring to a boil over medium heat. Reduce the heat and simmer until slightly thickened, 5 to 10 minutes. Add milk ¼ cup at a time if the sauce becomes too thick. Keep warm aside.

4. Meanwhile, bring a large pot of water to a boil over high heat. Cook the pasta according to the package directions until it is a little undercooked. Drain and add to the sauce. Add the reserved squash and peas, and stir until mixed.

5. Sprinkle the parsley on top. Serve hot.

Pesto Penne

Makes about 6 cups ■ *Ready in 30 minutes*

Chickpeas give this sauce a lovely creaminess. If you can use homemade almond milk, which doesn't take long to make, all the better.

8 ounces dried penne

2 cups broccoli florets in 1-inch pieces (about 6 ounces)

Leaves from 1½ bunches fresh basil (about 1½ packed cups)

2 to 3 small garlic cloves, coarsely chopped (about ½ tablespoon)

1 (15-ounce) can chickpeas, rinsed and drained (about 1½ cups)

1 cup Almond Milk (page 264) or unsweetened, unflavored store-bought

5 ounces cherry tomatoes, cut in half (about 1 cup)

Sea salt and freshly ground black pepper

Pinch of red pepper flakes (optional)

1. Bring a large saucepan of water to a boil over high heat. Cook the penne according to the package directions. Drain well and set aside.

2. Meanwhile, bring 2 cups water to a boil over medium-high heat in a small saucepan. Add the broccoli and cook over high heat for 5 minutes, until tender when pierced with a knife. Drain and set aside.

3. Place the basil, garlic, and ½ cup water in a blender. Blend until minced; do not puree the sauce completely. Set aside.

4. Place the chickpeas in a large saucepan and mash them using a masher, leaving the texture a little chunky; do not completely puree. (Alternatively, pulse in a food processor, then transfer to a large saucepan.) Add the almond milk and ½ cup water. Bring to a boil over medium heat.

5. Add the reserved basil and garlic mixture along with the tomatoes, salt and pepper to taste, and the red pepper flakes (if using). Reduce the heat and simmer until the flavors have blended and the tomatoes are slightly cooked and just beginning to soften, about 10 minutes.

6. Add the pasta and broccoli, and reheat
   over medium-low heat for 2 to 3 minutes.
   (Alternatively, pour the sauce over the pasta
   and broccoli.) Serve hot.

Storage: You can prepare the sauce, the broccoli, and
the pasta separately in advance and store them in airtight
containers in the refrigerator for up to 3 days. Combine and
cook everything just before serving, adding a little bit of water
to loosen the mixture.

Gnocchi Dokey

Makes about 1½ pounds (or 4 cups cooked) ▪ *Ready in 1½ hours*

Making homemade gnocchi is not complicated, and it's so much fun to do with kids, who love the experience of kneading and then rolling the dough into long "ropes" to be cut into individual pieces. Plus, the uncooked gnocchi freeze beautifully, so you can make a double batch and save half for another day. And let the kids take credit for making dinner!

1½ pounds Yukon Gold potatoes (about 3 medium), scrubbed

Sea salt

½ to ⅔ cup whole wheat flour, or as needed

3 cups Jimmy's Marinara Sauce (page 235), warmed, for serving

1. Preheat the oven to 400°F. Line a baking sheet with parchment paper.
2. Poke the potatoes with a knife four or five times and place them on the prepared baking sheet. Bake until very tender when poked with a fork, about 45 minutes, turning once or twice during baking.
3. Cool the potatoes until they can be handled. Peel off and discard the skins and place the flesh in a wide bowl. Mash until smooth using a ricer or a potato masher.
4. Add a few pinches of salt. Add the flour 1 tablespoon at a time while you knead the potatoes with your hands into a smooth, dry dough.
5. Divide the dough into four portions. On a clean, dry work surface, roll each portion into a ¾-inch-diameter rope. (Keep the remaining dough and dough ropes covered with a clean, dry kitchen towel to keep them from drying out.)
6. Cut each rope into ¾-inch-long pieces. Pinch each piece in the middle to create a dimple on

either side. As you work, transfer the gnocchi pieces to the baking sheet, keeping them in a single layer. (The gnocchi can be frozen at this point; see Storage.)

7. When ready to serve, bring a large stockpot of water to a boil over high heat. Drop about one-third of the gnocchi into the pot, one at a time. When they rise to the top, in 3 to 4 minutes, cook about 1 minute longer. Use a slotted spoon or spider to promptly transfer them to a platter without letting them touch one another (put a little water on the bottom of the platter if they are sticking).

8. Serve at once, topped with the warm marinara sauce.

Storage: The gnocchi can be prepared ahead through step 6 and put in the freezer on the baking sheet until frozen solid. Transfer them to a re-sealable bag and tightly seal. Store in the freezer for up to 1 month. When ready to cook, proceed as directed, cooking the gnocchi straight from the freezer; they may take a minute or two longer to cook.

RECIPES

Pad Thai–Style Noodles

Makes about 8 cups ■ *Ready in 30 minutes*

This tangy rice noodle and vegetable dish is a lighter and more flavorful riff on the standard pad Thai. The peanut sauce is light and very quick to make; if you want to make a double batch, you can store the extra in the refrigerator for up to a week and then mix it with vegetables and serve over steamed rice. To cut the prep time down even more, use a 16-ounce bag of your favorite frozen vegetable blend.

FOR THE PEANUT SAUCE

⅓ cup unsalted natural smooth peanut butter

¼ cup tomato paste

1 teaspoon garlic powder

1 teaspoon onion powder

1 teaspoon ground coriander

1 teaspoon dried lemon peel, or 2 teaspoons grated fresh zest

Pinch of cayenne pepper (optional)

Pinch of freshly ground black pepper

Sea salt

FOR THE PAD THAI

8 ounces Thai flat noodles

4 or 5 scallions, white and green parts, thinly sliced diagonally into 1-inch-long strips (about 1 cup)

2 (16-ounce) bags frozen stir-fry vegetables (about 8 cups)

6 small garlic cloves, minced (about 1 tablespoon)

1. Make the peanut sauce: In a blender or large bowl, place the peanut butter, tomato paste, garlic powder, onion powder, coriander, lemon peel, cayenne (if using), pepper, and 2 cups water. Blend or whisk until smooth. Set aside.

2. Make the pad Thai: Prepare the noodles according to the package directions. Drain, rinse with cold water if necessary, and drain again thoroughly.

3. In a large sauté pan, place the scallions, frozen vegetables, garlic, ginger, and ¼ cup water. Cover and cook over medium heat until the vegetables are tender, 5 to 10 minutes.

4. Add the spinach and the reserved peanut sauce to the vegetables and cook until the greens are wilted and the sauce thickens.

1 tablespoon grated fresh
   ginger

1 cup frozen or fresh baby
   spinach or chopped leaves

1 tablespoon finely chopped
   fresh Thai basil

1 tablespoon finely chopped
   fresh cilantro

1 lime, cut into wedges

5. Add the noodles to the vegetables. Mix well and cook over low heat until warmed through.

6. Garnish with the Thai basil and cilantro. Serve hot, with lime wedges on the side.

RECIPES

Chinese Noodles in Ginger Garlic Sauce 📷

Makes about 7 cups ■ *Ready in 25 minutes*

This quick and flavorful dish can be made quicker still by using frozen veggies in place of the fresh. Chow mein or lo mein Asian noodles are good here, but it's great with any other noodles, even spaghetti.

8 ounces dry lo mein or chow mein noodles, or any other long whole-grain noodles

3 tablespoons arrowroot powder

¼ cup low-sodium soy sauce or tamari

2 tablespoons brown rice vinegar

1½ tablespoons grated fresh ginger

9 small garlic cloves, minced (about 1½ tablespoons)

7 to 8 scallions, white and green parts, thinly sliced diagonally into 1-inch-long strips (about 2 cups)

8 ounces button mushrooms, trimmed and sliced (about 3 cups)

1 large carrot, thinly sliced (about 1 cup)

1½ cups broccoli florets in ½-inch pieces (about 5 ounces)

2 baby bok choy, trimmed and cut into 1-inch pieces (about 3 cups)

2 tablespoons finely chopped fresh cilantro

2 tablespoons cashews, toasted (see page 142) and chopped (optional)

1. Bring a large pot of water to a boil over high heat. Cook the noodles according to the package directions. Drain, rinse with cold water if necessary, and drain again thoroughly. Set aside.

2. In a medium bowl, mix the arrowroot powder, soy sauce, vinegar, and 1½ cups water until smooth. Set the slurry aside.

3. In a large sauté pan, place the ginger, garlic, scallions, mushrooms, carrot, and ¼ cup water. Cover and cook over medium heat until the vegetables are halfway cooked, about 5 minutes.

4. Add the broccoli and bok choy to the vegetables. Stir the reserved slurry and add it to the pan. Cover and cook until all the vegetables are crisp-tender and the sauce is slightly thickened, about 5 minutes.

5. Add the noodles to the vegetables; toss until well combined. Heat over medium-low heat if necessary to warm all the ingredients and add a little water to loosen the sauce, if necessary.

6. Garnish with the cilantro and cashews (if using) and serve hot.

Soba Noodle Salad

Makes about 6 cups ■ *Ready in 35 minutes*

With refreshing flavors of ginger, tamari, and toasted sesame seeds, this salad also showcases some unusual but very tasty vegetables. Burdock root has rich, earthy notes of artichokes, with some pungency. Arame is one of several kinds of sea vegetables that add a "from the sea" quality; its flavor is mild and a little sweet. Both of these, as well as the spicy daikon radish, can be found in Asian markets. You'll have some leftover burdock and daikon after making this salad; you can use them both in salads.

¼ cup arame or hijiki

6 ounces dry soba noodles

2 medium carrots, grated (about 1 cup)

¼ burdock root, washed, peeled, and grated (about ½ cup)

¼ daikon radish, peeled and grated (about ½ cup)

4 scallions, white and green parts, thinly sliced diagonally into 1-inch-long strips (about 1 cup)

1 tablespoon grated fresh ginger

3 tablespoons low-sodium tamari or soy sauce

2 tablespoons fresh lemon juice (from 1 lemon)

1 tablespoon roasted sesame seeds

Freshly ground black pepper

1. Place the arame in a small saucepan with 1 cup water. Soak for 20 minutes. Drain and return to the saucepan. Add 2 cups water and bring to a boil over medium-high heat. Boil for 5 minutes. Drain and set aside.

2. Bring a large saucepan of water to a boil over high heat. Cook the noodles according to the package directions. Drain. Rinse with cold water and drain again thoroughly. Transfer to a salad bowl.

3. In a skillet, place the carrots, burdock, daikon, scallions, ginger, and 2 tablespoons water. Cook over medium-low heat until the vegetables are slightly tender, 3 to 5 minutes, adding water 1 to 2 tablespoons at a time as needed to keep the vegetables from sticking.

4. In a small bowl, whisk together the tamari, lemon juice, sesame seeds, and pepper to taste. Pour over the noodles in the bowl. Add the sautéed vegetables and the reserved arame. Toss gently to combine. Serve warm or cold.

Udon Noodle Soup

Makes about 10 cups ■ Ready in 45 minutes

This very delicately flavored soup can be easily spiced up for more adventurous eaters by adding some extra black pepper. And you can increase the quantity or variety of vegetables without throwing off the balance at all.

6 ounces dry whole-grain udon noodles

8 ounces any type of fresh mushrooms, trimmed and thinly sliced (about 3 cups)

1 medium onion, thinly sliced (about 2 cups)

6 small garlic cloves, minced (about 1 tablespoon)

3 medium carrots, grated (about 1½ cups)

2 tablespoons low-sodium tamari or soy sauce

Sea salt and freshly ground black pepper

½ cup frozen green peas

2 scallions, white and green parts, thinly sliced (about ½ cup)

1. Bring a medium saucepan of water to a boil over high heat. Cook the noodles according to the package directions. Drain, rinse with cold water, and drain again thoroughly. Set aside.

2. Meanwhile, place the mushrooms, onion, garlic, and 4 cups water in a large saucepan. Cover and cook over medium heat until the mushrooms and onion are very tender, about 20 minutes.

3. Add the carrots, tamari, salt and pepper to taste, and 3 cups water to the broth. Bring to a boil over medium heat.

4. Stir in the reserved noodles along with the green peas and scallions. Bring to a boil over medium heat again. Serve hot.

AMAZING GRAINS

Couscous Bowls

Makes about 18 cups (about 8 bowls) ■ *Ready in 25 minutes*

This satisfying meal is equally good made with Israeli couscous or regular couscous. This recipe is a great jumping-off point for personal variations. Also feel free to use any other vegetables you like.

2 cups Vegetable Stock (page 262) or no-oil, low-sodium store-bought or water

½ teaspoon cumin seeds

2 cups dry whole wheat Israeli or regular couscous

Sea salt and freshly ground black pepper

1 medium head romaine lettuce, chopped into 1-inch pieces (9 to 10 cups)

2 small tomatoes, finely chopped (about 1 cup)

1 medium cucumber, finely chopped (about 1½ cups)

1 small red onion, thinly sliced (about 1 cup)

1 (15-ounce) can chickpeas, rinsed and drained (about 1½ cups)

2 tablespoons finely chopped fresh parsley

1 tablespoon fresh lemon juice (from ½ lemon)

Tahini Sauce (page 241)

1. In a small saucepan, bring the vegetable stock and cumin seeds to a boil over medium heat. Add the couscous and salt and pepper to taste. Return the stock to a boil, then cover the pan and remove from the heat. Let sit for 15 minutes, or until all the liquid is absorbed. Fluff with a fork.

2. To assemble eight bowls, in each one place some romaine lettuce, then the tomatoes, cucumber, onion, the couscous, and the chickpeas, dividing equally among the bowls.

3. Sprinkle with the parsley and lemon juice. Drizzle the tahini sauce on top. Serve at once.

Storage: For packed lunches, assemble the bowls directly in airtight containers. Let cool, then cover and refrigerate until ready to pack or serve.

RECIPES

RECIPES

Mexican Bowls ⬛ 📷

Makes about 12 cups (about 6 bowls) ■ *Ready in 45 minutes*

Rice and grain bowls are great for families. First, they're really filling. Plus, they're a fun "all hands on deck" meal, because kids of any age can help pull them together. There's chopping for the older kids and assembling for littler hands.

3 corn tortillas, cut into ¼-inch-thick strips (optional)

1 medium onion, thinly sliced (about 2 cups)

1 large zucchini, cut into 1-inch dice (about 2 cups)

1 red or green bell pepper, cored, seeded, and thinly sliced (about 2 cups)

3 cups cooked brown rice (from about ¾ cup dry)

Black Bean Spread (page 226)

2 cups shredded Savoy cabbage or romaine lettuce

1 medium tomato, finely chopped (about 1 cup)

4 scallions, white and green parts, thinly sliced (about 1 cup)

2 tablespoons finely chopped fresh cilantro

1 Hass avocado, pitted, peeled, and thinly sliced (about 1¼ cups)

2 tablespoons fresh lemon juice (from 1 lemon)

1. If tortilla strips are desired, preheat the oven to 350°F and line a baking sheet with parchment paper. Spread the corn tortilla strips on the prepared baking sheet. Bake until they are slightly brown and toasty, about 20 minutes. Set aside.

2. In a sauté pan, place the onion, zucchini, bell pepper, and ¼ cup water. Cook, covered, over medium heat until the onion is translucent, 5 to 10 minutes, adding water 1 to 2 tablespoons at a time to keep the vegetables from sticking.

3. Meanwhile, heat the brown rice and bean spread in separate small saucepans over low heat until hot; add water as needed to the bean spread to give it a more sauce-like consistency.

4. To assemble six bowls, divide the brown rice in the bottoms of the bowls and spoon some bean spread on top, dividing it evenly among the bowls. In this order, distribute the remaining

ingredients among the bowls: sautéed vegetables, shredded cabbage, tomato, scallions, cilantro, avocado, and tortilla strips.

5. Drizzle lemon juice on top of each bowl. Serve right away.

Storage: For packed lunches, assemble the bowls directly in airtight containers. Let cool, then cover and refrigerate until ready to pack or serve.

Tokyo Bowls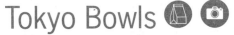

Makes about 16 cups (about 8 bowls) ■ *Ready in 45 minutes*

*This grain-based bowl has simple, mild flavors and fresh
ingredients—plus, it's quick to prepare. To bulk it up, add
some pickled root vegetables and canned beans.*

1 cup dry quinoa

1 cup dry millet

½ cup arame or hijiki
(optional)

1 pound sweet potatoes (about
2 medium), scrubbed and
cut into ¾-inch dice (about
4 cups)

2 large bunches kale, stems
removed, leaves chopped
into 1-inch pieces (about
14 cups)

3 cups mixed "California
Blend" frozen vegetables
(about 10 ounces)

2 cups Miso Lime Dressing
(page 245)

1. Place the quinoa and millet in a large bowl and
   fill it with water. Swish the grains around once
   or twice and then drain them. Repeat once
   more.

2. In a medium saucepan, bring 3½ cups water to
   a boil over medium-high heat. Add the drained
   millet and quinoa. Cover the pan and simmer
   for 20 minutes. Remove the pan from the heat
   and set aside, still covered, for 10 minutes.
   Uncover and fluff with a fork.

3. Meanwhile, if using the arame, place it in a
   small saucepan with 2 cups water. Soak for
   20 minutes. Drain and return to the saucepan.
   Add 4 cups water and bring to a boil over
   medium-high heat. Boil for 5 minutes. Drain and
   set aside.

4. Place a steamer basket in a sauté or saucepan,
   and add 1 to 2 inches of water. Cover and bring
   to a simmer. Place the sweet potatoes in the
   steamer, cover, and steam until tender when
   pierced with a fork but not mushy, 10 to 15
   minutes. Transfer the sweet potatoes to a large
   bowl to cool.

5. Place the kale and frozen vegetables in the steamer, cover, and steam until the kale has wilted, 3 to 5 minutes. Remove from the steamer and set aside.

6. To assemble eight bowls, divide the quinoa and millet among the bowls. In this order, distribute the remaining ingredients among the bowls: sweet potatoes, arame (if using), kale and vegetables.

7. Spoon the dressing on top. Serve hot.

Storage: For packed lunches, assemble the bowls directly in airtight containers. Let cool, then cover and refrigerate until ready to pack or serve.

RECIPES

Polenta Cubes and Roasted Vegetables with Barbecue Sauce

Makes about 4 cups polenta; about 4 cups roasted vegetables ∎ Ready in 1 hour 20 minutes

This dish is a big, satisfying meal that looks and tastes gourmet. You can make the polenta and the sauce a day in advance, so all you have to do is reheat and serve.

5 cups Vegetable Stock (page 262) or no-oil, low-sodium store-bought or water

1 cup dry polenta

½ teaspoon ground turmeric

Sea salt and freshly ground black pepper

2 medium zucchini, sliced diagonally ¼ inch thick (about 3 cups)

2 small portobello mushrooms, stemmed and cut into ½-inch-wide strips (about 3 cups)

1 medium onion, cut into ¼-inch wedges (about 2 cups)

2 large carrots, sliced diagonally 1 inch thick (about 1½ cups)

1 large Japanese eggplant, cut into 2 x ½-inch strips (about 3 cups)

2 cups Barbecue Sauce (with chipotle if desired, page 238), or oil-free store-bought

2 tablespoons finely chopped fresh parsley

1. Bring the vegetable stock to a boil over medium-high heat in a large saucepan. While whisking constantly, add the polenta in a slow and steady stream. Break up any clumps. Add the turmeric and salt and pepper to taste. Simmer, stirring frequently, until all the stock is absorbed and the polenta is cooked, 20 to 25 minutes.

2. Pour the hot polenta at once into an 8-inch square pan and smooth the top. Let cool for 20 to 30 minutes, until the polenta is firm.

3. Meanwhile, preheat the oven to 425°F. Line two baking sheets with parchment paper.

4. Arrange the zucchini, mushrooms, onion, carrots, and eggplant in single layers on the prepared baking sheets. Bake for 20 minutes. Stir the vegetables and bake until tender, another 20 minutes. Remove from the oven and cover to keep warm. (The polenta and vegetables can be refrigerated at this point; see Storage.)

5. Reduce the oven temperature to 350°F.

6. Cut the cooled polenta into 2-inch squares. Use a spatula to move them around so there is space between the squares. Bake the polenta until warmed through, about 20 minutes.

7. Meanwhile, heat the barbecue sauce in a small saucepan over low heat.

8. For each serving, place one or two squares of polenta on a plate, top with the roasted vegetables, and pour some barbecue sauce over the vegetables. Garnish with parsley. Serve at once, passing the remaining barbecue sauce on the side.

Storage: The polenta and vegetables can be prepared ahead of time through step 4. Cover the polenta with plastic wrap and transfer the vegetables to an airtight container. Refrigerate both for up to 1 day. When ready to serve, preheat the oven to 350°F. Cut the polenta as directed, then reheat both the polenta and the roasted vegetables until hot.

RECIPES

Jambalaya

Makes about 14 cups ■ Ready in 1 hour

This variation on the classic Louisiana dish is a great and oh-so-flavorful one-pot meal with beans, vegetables, rice, and lots of spice (which naturally you can adjust according to your taste).

1 small onion, cut into ¼-inch dice (about 1 cup)

1 green bell pepper, cored, seeded, and cut into ¼-inch dice (about 1 cup)

1 red bell pepper, cored, seeded, and cut into ¼-inch dice (about 1 cup)

2 large celery stalks, cut into ¼-inch pieces (about 1 cup)

6 small garlic cloves, minced (about 1 tablespoon)

3 dried bay leaves

2 cups dry brown rice

3 cups Vegetable Stock (page 262) or no-oil, low-sodium store-bought or water, as needed

1 medium tomato, cut into ¼-inch dice (about 1 cup)

1 tablespoon vegan Worcestershire sauce

1 teaspoon hot sauce, or to taste (optional)

1. In a large stew pot or Dutch oven, place the onion, bell peppers, celery, garlic, bay leaves, and ½ cup water. Cover and cook over medium heat until the onion is translucent, about 10 minutes, adding water 1 tablespoon at a time as needed to keep the vegetables from sticking.

2. Add the rice, stock, tomato, Worcestershire sauce, hot sauce (if using), and Creole seasoning. Bring the stock to a boil over medium heat. Reduce the heat, cover, and simmer for 20 minutes, until the rice is half cooked, stirring occasionally and adding more stock or water as needed to prevent sticking.

3. Add the tomato paste, chickpeas, beans, and lemon juice. Stir in ½ cup water and add salt and pepper to taste. Mix well, cover, and cook until the liquid is absorbed and the rice is completely cooked, about 25 minutes.

¼ cup Mild Creole Seasoning
(page 169) or store-bought

1 (6-ounce) can no-salt-added
tomato paste (about ⅔ cup)

1 (15-ounce) can chickpeas,
rinsed and drained (about
1½ cups)

1 (15-ounce) can red kidney
beans, rinsed and drained
(about 1½ cups)

1 tablespoon fresh lemon juice
(from ½ lemon)

Sea salt and freshly ground
black pepper

1 tablespoon finely chopped
fresh parsley

4. Taste and adjust the seasoning. Remove and discard the bay leaves. Garnish with the parsley. Serve hot.

Corn and Tomato Risotto

Makes about 5 cups ■ *Ready in 1 hour*

*This delectable risotto gets its creaminess from the almond milk
and nutritional yeast, and a nice crunch from the corn.*

1 cup dry short-grain brown rice, rinsed and drained

1 small onion, finely chopped (about 1 cup)

6 small garlic cloves, minced (about 1 tablespoon)

2 to 3 cups Vegetable Stock (page 262) or no-oil, low-sodium store-bought, or as needed

1 medium tomato, finely chopped (about 1 cup)

1 cup frozen or fresh corn kernels

4 ounces oyster or other wild mushrooms, sliced (about 1 cup)

1 teaspoon dried marjoram

1 teaspoon dried thyme

½ cup Almond Milk (page 264) or unsweetened, unflavored store-bought

1 tablespoon red wine vinegar, or to taste

2 tablespoons nutritional yeast

¼ cup chopped fresh chives, or 2 tablespoons dried

Sea salt and freshly ground black pepper

1. In a sauté pan, place the rice, onion, garlic, and 2 cups of the stock. Bring to a boil over medium-high heat, then reduce the heat and simmer for 25 minutes, until the rice is half cooked.

2. Stir in the tomato, corn, mushrooms, marjoram, and thyme and cook until the rice is tender, about 25 minutes, stirring frequently and adding more stock if needed.

3. Add the almond milk, vinegar, nutritional yeast, chives, and salt and pepper to taste. Cook until creamy, about 10 minutes. Serve hot.

RECIPES

Quinoa Pilaf

Makes about 5 cups ■ *Ready in 45 minutes*

This recipe is a take on vegetable pulao, *a traditional Indian rice pilaf,
made here with quinoa and tarragon, an herb that is not common
in Indian cooking but that adds a sweet aromatic quality.*

2 cups Vegetable Stock
(page 262) or no-oil,
low-sodium store-bought

1 cup dry quinoa, washed and
drained

½ leek, white and light green
parts only, finely chopped
(about ½ cup)

½ cup cauliflower florets
in ½-inch pieces (about
1½ ounces)

1 medium carrot, cut into
¼-inch dice (about ½ cup)

3 ounces green beans,
trimmed and cut into ¼-inch
pieces (about ½ cup)

1 small garlic clove, minced
(about ½ teaspoon)

1 teaspoon dried tarragon,
or ½ teaspoon fresh

1 or 2 dried bay leaves

Sea salt and freshly ground
black pepper

¾ cup frozen green peas

1 tablespoon fresh lemon juice
(from ½ lemon)

2 tablespoons finely chopped
fresh cilantro or parsley

1. In a small saucepan, bring the vegetable stock
   to a boil over medium-high heat. Cover and
   keep hot.

2. Toast the quinoa in a medium saucepan over
   medium-low heat until it is completely dry and
   lightly brown, 5 to 10 minutes. Stir frequently to
   keep it from burning.

3. Add the hot stock to the quinoa along with the
   leek, cauliflower, carrot, green beans, garlic,
   tarragon, bay leaves, and salt and pepper to
   taste.

4. Bring the liquid to a boil over medium heat.
   Reduce the heat, cover the pan, and simmer
   for 20 minutes.

5. Meanwhile, place the frozen green peas in a
   colander and run cold water over them to thaw.
   Drain well and set aside.

6. Remove the pilaf from the heat. Fluff the
   quinoa with a fork and gently mix in the peas
   and the lemon juice. Cover and let sit for 10 to
   15 minutes. Remove and discard the bay leaves.

7. Sprinkle with the cilantro or parsley and
   serve hot.

RECIPES

Samosa Stuffed Muffins 🔺

Makes 12 muffins ■ *Ready in 1 hour*

Samosas, which are fried or baked dumplings filled with aromatic vegetables, are a staple of Indian cuisine and for good reason: they are delicious. But they are also time-consuming to prepare, especially when trying to keep them oil-free. These muffins, on the other hand, have the delicious flavor and aroma of traditional samosas, but they take much less time and are much easier to make. They are especially good served with Cilantro Lime Chutney (page 239). These muffins are nice in a packed lunch or for a party, so you may want to make a double batch.

FOR THE STUFFING
1 teaspoon cumin seeds
1 large potato (about
   ¾ pound), scrubbed and
   cut into ½-inch dice (about
   3 cups)
1 small onion, thinly sliced
   (about 1 cup)
6 small garlic cloves, minced
   (about 1 tablespoon)
A 2-inch piece jalapeño
   pepper, seeded and
   finely chopped (about
   1 tablespoon; optional)
½ teaspoon ground turmeric
1 tablespoon finely chopped
   fresh cilantro
Pinch of cayenne pepper
   (optional)
Sea salt and freshly ground
   black pepper

FOR THE MUFFINS
1 cup all-purpose flour
1 cup fine cornmeal
1 tablespoon ground flaxseed
1 tablespoon baking powder

1. Preheat the oven to 350°F. Line a standard muffin pan with cupcake liners.

2. Make the filling: In a sauté pan, toast the cumin seeds over medium heat, until slightly brown and aromatic, 2 to 3 minutes. Add the potato, onion, garlic, jalapeño, turmeric, and ½ cup water. Cover the pan and cook over medium heat until the potato is tender when pierced with a fork, 7 to 10 minutes, adding water 1 tablespoon at a time as needed to keep the vegetables from sticking.

3. Stir in the cilantro, cayenne pepper (if using), and salt and pepper to taste. Mix well. Remove from the heat and let cool.

4. Make the muffins: In a large bowl, whisk together the flour, cornmeal, flaxseed, baking powder, salt, and pepper.

5. In a separate bowl, whisk together the milk, sesame paste, and vinegar.

½ teaspoon sea salt

Pinch of freshly ground black pepper

1½ cups unsweetened, unflavored plant milk

¼ cup sesame seed paste (tahini)

2 teaspoons apple cider vinegar

1½ cups Cilantro Lime Chutney (page 239), for serving

6. Add the liquid ingredients to the dry ingredients and stir together with a wooden spoon until well mixed.

7. Spoon a rounded tablespoon of batter in each cup of the muffin pan. Divide the stuffing evenly among the cups. Spoon the remaining batter on top.

8. Bake until a toothpick inserted in the middle of a muffin comes out clean, 35 to 45 minutes.

9. Remove the pan from the oven and place on a rack to cool for a few minutes. Unmold the muffins and serve warm with the chutney.

Storage: Store in an airtight container at room temperature for up to 1 day, in the refrigerator for up to 3 days, or in the freezer for up to 1 month.

RECIPES

RECIPES

7 Grain Bread

Makes 2 (8½ × 4½-inch) loaves ■ *Ready in 3 hours*

Baking your own bread may not be an everyday thing, but on a day when you have the time, the process is so satisfying, and it's a great activity to do with kids. They love the feel of the fresh dough as much as adults do. Plus, there's nothing that compares to the taste and aroma of freshly baked bread. This recipe makes two loaves so you can freeze one for later.

5 cups whole wheat flour, plus more for dusting

2 (¼-ounce) packages active dry yeast (4½ teaspoons)

2 cups lukewarm (110°F to 115°F) tap water

2 tablespoons Date Paste (page 265) or pure maple syrup

¼ cup dry quinoa (optional)

¼ cup dry millet (optional)

¼ cup dry amaranth (optional)

2 cups boiling water (optional)

1 cup mixed-grain flour (see Note)

1½ teaspoons sea salt (optional)

2 tablespoons old-fashioned rolled oats

2 tablespoons flaxseeds

1 teaspoon caraway seeds (optional)

1. Line two 8½ × 4½-inch loaf pans with parchment paper. Dust the bottoms with some flour.

2. In a large bowl, mix 2 cups of the flour, the yeast, and the lukewarm water until well combined. Add the date paste and very lightly stir it in. Cover with a cloth and set in a warm place, such as by the stove or in a warm oven, until the sponge starts to rise, about 30 minutes.

3. Meanwhile, in a small bowl, combine the quinoa, millet, and amaranth (if using). Pour the boiling water (if using) over the grains. Cover and let stand for 30 minutes. Drain thoroughly in a fine-mesh strainer.

4. Transfer the sponge and drained grains (if using) to a food processor fitted with a dough blade. Add the remaining 3 cups flour, the mixed-grain flour, and the salt (if using). (The bowl may be very full, but the mixture will shrink when it comes together.) Process the mixture 3 to 5 minutes, until it forms a cohesive dough.

5. Transfer the dough to the large bowl. Cover with a damp cloth and let rise in a warm place for 60 minutes, until the dough has doubled.

6. Dust a clean work surface with some flour and transfer the dough to it. Knead with your hands, adding more flour as necessary, until the dough is smooth.

7. Divide the dough into two equal portions. Shape each portion into a loaf and place in the loaf pans. Brush the tops with some water. Sprinkle with the oats, flaxseeds, and caraway seeds (if using).

8. Cover each pan with a damp cloth and let rise in a warm place for 20 minutes, until the dough doubles in size. Preheat the oven to 375°F.

9. Bake 30 to 35 minutes or until the loaves are golden and firm to the touch and the internal temperature registers between 190°F and 205°F on an instant-read thermometer.

10. Cool the loaves in the pans for 5 to 10 minutes, then unmold and peel off the parchment paper. Let cool completely on racks.

Storage: Wrap bread tightly and store at room temperature for 5 to 7 days or freeze for up to 2 months.

Note: To make the mixed-grain flour, combine at least three of these flours in any proportion to make 1 cup: rye, barley, rice, buckwheat, quinoa, sorghum, oat, cornmeal, or spelt. You can use just a few or all of them to make a less dense, less wheaty bread.

Cornbread 📷

Makes 1 (9-inch square) bread ■ Ready in 1 hour

This cornbread is moist and crumbly and delicious. Serve it with soup or stew.

1 tablespoon flaxseeds

1 cup frozen corn kernels, coarsely crushed in a food processor or blender

1 cup unsweetened, unflavored plant milk

¼ cup Date Paste (page 265) or pure maple syrup

1 cup whole wheat flour

1¼ cups coarse cornmeal

½ cup almond flour

2 tablespoons dried chives, or ¼ tablespoon chopped fresh (optional)

1 tablespoon dried parsley, or 2 tablespoons chopped fresh (optional)

2 teaspoons baking powder

¼ teaspoon baking soda

½ teaspoon sea salt, or to taste

½ tablespoon sesame seeds

1. Preheat the oven to 350°F. Line a 9-inch square deep baking dish with parchment paper.

2. In a small saucepan, place the flaxseeds and 1 cup water. Bring to a boil over medium-high heat. Reduce the heat and simmer for 1 to 2 minutes.

3. Strain the liquid into a glass measuring cup; discard the seeds and reserve ¾ cup of the liquid.

4. In a medium bowl, place the corn, milk, date paste, and the reserved flax cooking liquid. Whisk until well blended.

5. In a large bowl, whisk together the wheat flour, cornmeal, almond flour, chives and parsley (if using), baking powder, baking soda, and salt until well blended.

6. Make a well in the middle of the dry ingredients. Pour the liquid into the well. Use a wooden spoon to mix quickly and gently to form a batter.

7. Pour the batter into the baking dish. Sprinkle the sesame seeds on top.

8. Bake until a toothpick inserted in the middle of the cornbread comes out dry, 40 to 50 minutes. Remove to a rack to cool in the pan for 5 or 10 minutes. Unmold and peel off the parchment paper. Let cool completely on the rack. Cut while warm or once cooled into squares.

Storage: Wrap tightly and keep refrigerated for 4 to 5 days.

Tomatillo Sauce over Potatoes

Makes 1 (9 × 13-inch) casserole ■ Ready in 30 minutes

This dish came about by accident, as so many quick meals do. I needed to whip up a dish for an unplanned dinner party, and I had some baked potatoes and tomatillo sauce in the fridge, so I decided to bake them together. It turned out to be such a hit with the guests that it became a regular in my rotation of quick-and-easy recipes.

2 pounds russet potatoes (about 4 medium), baked (see Note)

2 to 3 cups fresh or frozen green peas and/or corn kernels

Tomatillo Sauce (page 240)

2 tablespoons finely chopped fresh cilantro

1. Preheat the oven to 350°F.
2. Cut the potatoes into 1- to 1½-inch pieces and place them in a 9 × 13-inch casserole. Add the peas and/or corn and stir gently to combine. Pour as much of the tomatillo sauce over the potatoes and peas and/or corn as is necessary to cover them.
3. Bake 20 minutes, until heated through and the sauce bubbles. Garnish with the cilantro and serve hot, passing any remaining tomatillo sauce on the side.

Note: If you're not using leftover baked potatoes, place scrubbed uncooked potatoes on a baking sheet and bake in a 400°F oven for 40 minutes, or until soft when poked with a fork.

RECIPES

Quick Hummus and Quinoa Wraps

Makes 4 wraps ▪ Ready in 15 minutes

If you're staring at a bunch of leftovers in the fridge and can't figure out how to turn them into a meal, let this recipe be your guide. You can quickly transform those leftovers into tasty wraps for dinner or lunch boxes. All you need for your base are whole wheat tortillas and any of the spreads or hummus in this book (pages 224 to 225), or use your favorite oil-free store-bought spread. Then let your imagination soar: a cooked grain adds heft and whatever raw or sautéed veggies you have add crunch.

4 whole wheat tortillas

2 cups Sesame-Seed Hummus (page 227) or other spread

1 cup cooked quinoa or other grain

2 cups fresh spinach

2 medium tomatoes, thinly sliced (about 2 cups)

1. Warm the tortillas one at a time for about 20 seconds on each side in a dry skillet set over medium heat. Or if you have a gas stove, place a tortilla straight over the flame for a few seconds on each side. As you remove each one from the pan, stack them and cover with a damp cloth to keep them from getting crisp.
2. Place 1 tortilla on a clean work surface. Spread with a layer of hummus, then top with some of the quinoa, spinach, and tomatoes. Tightly roll up the tortilla and place on a plate or platter.
3. Repeat with the remaining tortillas and fillings. Keep tightly in place so that they stay rolled. Serve.

Storage: Wrap each wrap tightly in wax paper for up to 2 days in the refrigerator.

Marinated Tempeh 🔲

Makes 6 to 8 slices ■ *Ready in 25 minutes (plus 30 minutes for marinating)*

When a dish calls for just part of a package of tempeh, as is the case with the Polenta Tempeh Casserole (page 178), it can be hard to know what to do with the remainder. I like this quick solution, and the result makes a great light dinner or bagged lunch the day after. Proportions are based on half a package, but, of course, you can prepare a full package—or any quantity— this way. Just increase or decrease the dipping sauce proportionally.

4 ounces tempeh (half an 8-ounce package)

½ cup Tamari Sesame Dipping Sauce (page 228), or as needed

Ranch Dressing (page 242) or other sauce, for serving

1. Slice the tempeh ¼ inch thick and lay the slices in a single layer in a shallow dish. Pour the dipping sauce over the top. Turn the slices to thoroughly coat them and set aside for 30 minutes.

2. Heat a nonstick skillet over medium heat. Remove the tempeh from the marinade and let the excess drip off. Add to the pan and toast for about 20 minutes, until brown on both sides, turning once or twice.

3. Serve with ranch dressing or your favorite sauce.

Storage: Store in an airtight container in the refrigerator for up to 3 days.

RECIPES

Quick Black Bean Tostadas

Makes 10 tostadas ■ *Ready in 30 minutes*

Toasted, crispy tortillas topped with savory ingredients, known as tostadas across Latin America, are delicious as a snack or light meal. They can be prepared very quickly when the tortillas are toasted in advance (they'll stay crisp for as long as a couple of weeks, depending on the humidity where you live), and they can be a great way to use up leftovers you have in the fridge. Black bean spread is a good base to hold other ingredients, but you can use any kind of thick dip or spread, or even mashed potatoes or avocado.

10 corn tortillas

Black Bean Spread (page 226)

1 small tomato, finely chopped (about ½ cup)

3 scallions, white and green parts, thinly sliced (about ¾ cup)

½ small head romaine lettuce, finely shredded (about 2 cups)

2 to 3 tablespoons finely chopped fresh cilantro

1. Preheat the oven to 350°F.
2. Arrange the tortillas in a single layer on a rimmed baking sheet.
3. Toast in the oven until crisp, about 20 minutes.
4. Meanwhile, warm the black bean spread in a small saucepan over low heat.
5. Spread about ¼ cup bean spread on each tortilla. Sprinkle on the tomato, scallions, romaine lettuce, and cilantro. Serve at once.

Storage: The tortillas can be toasted in advance. Store in an airtight container at room temperature for up to 2 weeks.

Savory Quick Oats with Veggies

Makes about 2½ cups ■ Ready in 10 to 15 minutes

Oats aren't often considered a meal outside of breakfast, but when mixed with vegetables and hot sauce, they are a fantastic lunch, afternoon snack, or even late-night supper. I keep quick oats in my pantry specifically for such occasions. Old-fashioned rolled oats can also be used; they just take longer to cook and require more liquid (follow the guidelines on the package).

1 teaspoon garlic powder
½ teaspoon dried oregano
1 cup quick oats
1 cup frozen mixed vegetables
1 medium tomato, cut into
   ½-inch dice (about 1 cup)
1 cup fresh or frozen spinach
1 tablespoon fresh lemon juice
   (from ½ lemon)
A few dashes of hot sauce, or
   to taste (optional)
Sea salt and freshly ground
   black pepper

1. In a medium saucepan, place 1½ cups water, garlic powder, and oregano and bring to a boil over medium-high heat. Stir in the oats and simmer until they begin to soften, about 2 minutes.

2. Add the frozen vegetables, tomato, spinach, lemon juice, hot sauce (if using), and salt and pepper to taste. Cook, uncovered, until the vegetables are cooked and the greens are wilted, 5 to 7 minutes. Serve hot.

RECIPES

RECIPES

Quick Mediterranean Pizzas

Makes 2 (12-inch) pizzas ■ *Ready in 30 minutes*

These pizzas are quickly made from store-bought pizza crust (or frozen homemade; see pages 18 and 266) and leftovers such as bean spread or cheesy sauce and marinara sauce. Adding some veggies on top gives them a great color and makes them into a hearty, satisfying meal.

2 (12-inch) no-oil, store-bought pizza crusts

1 cup Jimmy's Marinara Sauce (page 235) or store-bought

3 cups frozen Mediterranean blend vegetables, such as green beans, summer squash, red peppers, carrots, and onions (about 12 ounces)

2 cups White Bean Rosemary Dip (page 224) or Yukon Golden Cheese (page 233)

¼ cup chopped black olives (optional)

2 tablespoons nutritional yeast

Sea salt

Red pepper flakes (optional)

1. Preheat the oven to 400°F. Line two baking sheets with parchment paper.

2. Place the pizza crusts on the prepared baking sheets. Spread the marinara sauce on top, dividing it equally between the crusts and leaving an uncovered border around the edge.

3. Spread the vegetables evenly on each pizza and spoon the bean dip or cheese sauce on top.

4. Sprinkle the olives (if using) and the nutritional yeast on top of each, followed by a little salt to taste and some red pepper flakes (if using).

5. Bake for about 20 minutes until the crust edges are brown and crispy. Slice and serve hot.

Storage: Tightly wrap leftover pizza in wax paper and store in the refrigerator for up to 2 days. Reheat in a preheated 350°F oven for 20 minutes.

Quick Noodle Soup

Makes about 6 cups ■ *Ready in 25 minutes*

Noodles and frozen vegetables are kitchen staples that can be whipped up into a soup dinner in minutes. You can use stock instead of water, but it's not necessary when you add a flavorful spice blend. Some great choices for this tasty soup are Mild Creole Seasoning (page 169) or store-bought Creole seasoning, or Thai or Moroccan seasoning mixes.

5 cups water or Vegetable Stock (page 262) or low-sodium store-bought

2 scallions, white and green parts, thinly sliced (about ½ cup)

6 small garlic cloves, minced (about 1 tablespoon)

1 tablespoon grated fresh ginger

1 tablespoon spice blend of choice

4 ounces dry Thai or other rice noodles

1 (16-ounce) bag frozen stir-fry vegetables (about 4 cups)

2 tablespoons fresh lemon or lime juice (from 1 lemon or lime)

1 tablespoon no-salt-added tomato paste (optional)

Sea salt

1 tablespoon finely chopped fresh cilantro (optional)

1. In a large saucepan, place the water, scallions, garlic, ginger, and spice blend. Cover and bring to a boil over medium heat.

2. Add the noodles and simmer for about 5 minutes, or until the noodles are halfway cooked.

3. Add the frozen vegetables, lemon juice, and tomato paste (if using).

4. Cook until the vegetables are tender and the noodles are al dente or cooked as desired. Add salt to taste. Garnish with the cilantro (if using), and serve hot.

Quick Mushroom Risotto

Makes about 6 cups ■ *Ready in 20 minutes*

*It's surprising how quickly you can make a tasty risotto
when you have leftover gravy and cooked rice.*

4 cups cooked brown rice (from about 1 cup dry)

3 cups Cremini Mushroom Gravy (page 236)

2 cups frozen mixed vegetables, such as green peas, carrots, and green beans

1 tablespoon white wine vinegar

2 teaspoons garlic powder

2 tablespoons nutritional yeast

1. In a large saucepan, place the rice, gravy, frozen vegetables, vinegar, and garlic powder. Cook over medium-low heat until the vegetables are cooked, and the texture is creamy, 10 to 15 minutes.

2. Stir in the nutritional yeast until well blended. Serve hot.

RECIPES

Rice and Bean Salad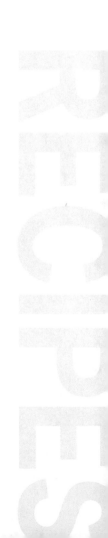

Makes about 3 cups ■ *Ready in 10 minutes*

For a more filling salad, add a few cups of lightly cooked frozen vegetables.

**2 cups cooked brown rice
or any other grain (from
½ to ⅔ cup dry), cooled**

**1 (15-ounce) can black beans
or other variety, rinsed and
drained (about 1½ cups)**

**1 cup Pico de Gallo
(page 230) or store-bought**

**1 small head romaine lettuce,
trimmed and shredded
(about 4 cups)**

**Sea salt and freshly ground
black pepper**

In a large bowl, place the rice, beans, pico de gallo, romaine lettuce, and salt and pepper to taste. Mix well. Taste and adjust the seasoning. Serve at once or chill and serve cold.

Storage: Store in an airtight container in the refrigerator for up to 3 days.

DIPS, SPREADS, SAUCES, AND DRESSINGS

White Bean Rosemary Dip

Makes about 3 cups ▪ Ready in 20 minutes (plus 20 minutes for chilling)

This creamy dip is good served with crudités or chips, as well as a spread in sandwiches, stuffed pitas, and wraps such as the Vegetable Breakfast Quesadilla (page 100). If using home-cooked beans, make sure they are very well cooked and tender in order to get the creamiest texture.

2 (15-ounce) cans white beans, rinsed and drained (about 3 cups)

½ red bell pepper, cored, seeded, and finely chopped (about ½ cup)

½ small onion, finely chopped (about ½ cup)

3 small garlic cloves, minced (about ½ tablespoon)

2 tablespoons fresh lime juice (from 1 lime)

1 teaspoon dried rosemary

½ jalapeño pepper, cored, seeded, and minced (optional)

Sea salt and freshly ground black pepper

1. In a medium saucepan, place the white beans, bell pepper, onion, garlic, lime juice, rosemary, jalapeño (if using), and ¼ cup water. Bring to a simmer over medium heat. Simmer until the onion is translucent, 5 to 10 minutes.

2. Remove from the heat and mash the mixture with a hand masher or pulse in a food processor, keeping the texture a bit coarse. Add salt and pepper to taste. Chill for about 20 minutes. Serve.

Storage: Store in an airtight container in the refrigerator for up to 3 days.

Cheesy Dressing

Makes about 3½ cups ■ *Ready in 30 minutes*

This versatile sauce is excellent tossed with veggies or with chips, pita bread, and anything else you or your kids like to dip. You can also mix leftover sauce with warm cooked pasta for a quick mac 'n cheese, or use it as a cheesy spread in wraps and sandwiches. It's a good standby for packed lunches with celery or carrot sticks. White miso is fermented for a shorter period than other varieties of miso and therefore is milder and less salty. It contributes to the cheesy flavor. The optional turmeric adds nice color.

1 pound trimmed cauliflower, cut into 1-inch florets (about 5 cups)

½ pound Yukon Gold potato (about 1 medium), cut into ½-inch dice (about 2 cups)

2 small garlic cloves

⅛ teaspoon ground turmeric (optional)

½ cup nutritional yeast

2 teaspoons white wine vinegar

½ teaspoon dried marjoram

½ teaspoon mild white miso (optional)

¼ teaspoon prepared yellow mustard

Sea salt and freshly ground black or white pepper

½ cup unsweetened, unflavored plant-based milk, or as needed

1. In a large saucepan, place the cauliflower, potato, garlic, turmeric (if using), and 1 cup water. Bring to a boil over medium heat, then reduce the heat and simmer until the vegetables are very tender, about 10 minutes. Remove the pan from the heat and set aside just until very warm, but not piping hot.

2. Transfer the cauliflower mixture with all its liquid to a blender. Add the nutritional yeast, vinegar, marjoram, miso (if using), mustard, and salt and pepper to taste. Blend until creamy and smooth, adding milk as necessary to achieve the desired consistency. Serve at once.

Storage: Store in an airtight container in the refrigerator for 3 to 4 days. To reheat, place in a saucepan and stir in some milk or water to loosen, then heat over medium-low heat until hot.

RECIPES

Black Bean Spread

Makes about 2½ cups ■ *Ready in 15 minutes*

*Serve this quick-to-make and always satisfying spread in a flat dish
topped with fresh cilantro, as well as diced tomatoes and avocado,
if desired, for a very pretty presentation. It's tasty with tortilla
chips and with rice and veggies in the Mexican Bowls (page 200),
as well as in the Quick Black Bean Tostadas (page 218).*

2 (15-ounce) cans black
beans, rinsed and drained
(about 3 cups)

1½ tablespoons onion powder

1½ tablespoons garlic powder

1 teaspoon ground cumin

2 tablespoons fresh lemon
juice (from 1 lemon)

Sea salt and freshly ground
black pepper

1 tablespoon finely chopped
fresh cilantro

1. In a medium saucepan, stir together the beans, onion powder, garlic powder, cumin, lemon juice, and salt and pepper to taste; add ½ cup water. Cook over medium heat until the flavors have blended, about 10 minutes. Add more water if needed to keep the beans from sticking to the bottom of the pan.

2. Remove the pan from the heat and use a potato masher to mash the beans to the desired texture. If you prefer a creamier texture, add more water as you mash. Taste and adjust the seasoning.

3. Transfer to a flat serving bowl and serve warm, or chill and serve cold. Garnish with the cilantro just before serving.

Storage: Store in an airtight container in the refrigerator for 3 to 4 days. To reheat, place in a medium saucepan with a small amount of water and heat over low heat until warm, stirring frequently to prevent sticking.

Sesame-Seed Hummus

Makes about 2 cups ■ *Ready in 35 minutes*

Tahini, a smooth paste made from roasted sesame seeds, is included in most recipes for hummus. It's delicious, but can make the resulting chickpea dip a little heavy. This easy-to-make hummus has a much lighter and fluffier texture than regular hummus thanks to the use of raw sesame seeds instead of tahini.

¼ cup sesame seeds

1 (15-ounce) can chickpeas, rinsed and drained (about 1½ cups)

3 small garlic cloves

3 tablespoons fresh lime juice (from 1½ limes)

Sea salt and freshly ground black pepper

1 tablespoon finely chopped fresh parsley (optional)

1. Place the sesame seeds in a small bowl and cover with ½ cup water. Soak for 30 minutes.
2. Pour the seeds and soaking water into a blender and blend into a smooth paste.
3. Add the chickpeas, garlic, lime juice, and salt and pepper to taste. Blend until smooth.
4. Add the parsley (if using) and pulse until evenly mixed. Serve.

Storage: Store in an airtight container in the refrigerator for 4 to 5 days.

Tamari Sesame Dipping Sauce

Makes about ⅔ cup ▪ Ready in 15 minutes

This sauce comes together really quickly, and it can be stored in the fridge for up to one week. Make a double batch and keep it around as a salad dressing or as a dipping sauce for Fresh Vegetable Temaki Rolls (page 124), spring rolls, pot stickers, or in place of the miso lime dressing in the Tokyo Bowls (page 202).

2 tablespoons fresh lime juice (from 1 lime)

1 tablespoon low-sodium tamari or soy sauce

1 tablespoon Date Paste (page 265)

1 teaspoon grated fresh ginger

2 small cloves garlic, minced (about 1 teaspoon)

Pinch of ground white pepper or red pepper flakes

½ teaspoon black or white sesame seeds

1. In a jar with a tight-fitting lid, place ⅓ cup water and the lime juice, tamari, date paste, ginger, garlic, and pepper. Close tightly and shake well.

2. Toast the sesame seeds in a dry skillet over medium-low heat, shaking the pan often, until black seeds start to crackle and pop or white seeds are lightly browned, about 5 minutes. Add to the jar and shake to combine. Use at once or chill until ready to serve.

Storage: Store in the tightly closed jar in the refrigerator for up to 10 days.

Sweet Salsa Fresca

Makes about 4 cups ■ *Ready in 10 minutes*

*This quick recipe for fresh salsa makes a great accompaniment
to Vegetable Breakfast Quesadillas (page 100), and is also good
served with chips. Use any seasonal fruit; some of my favorites
here are mangoes, pineapples, peaches, grapes, and pears.*

**1 cup diced seasonal fresh
fruit in ¼-inch pieces**

**1 medium apple, any variety,
cored and cut into ¼-inch
dice (about 1 cup)**

**1 large tomato, cored,
seeded, and cut into ¼-inch
dice (about 1½ cups)**

**½ small onion, cut into ¼-inch
dice (about ½ cup)**

**½ jalapeño or serrano pepper,
seeded and minced (about
2 tablespoons; optional)**

**¼ cup finely chopped fresh
cilantro**

**2 tablespoons fresh lemon
juice (from 1 lemon)**

Sea salt (optional)

In a large bowl, mix the fruit, apple, tomato, onion,
jalapeño (if using), cilantro, and lemon juice.
Keep refrigerated until ready to serve. Add salt (if
using) to taste just before serving.

Storage: Store in an airtight container in the refrigerator for up
to 2 days.

Pico de Gallo

Makes about 3 cups ■ *Ready in 10 minutes*

A classic for a reason, this quickly prepared salsa can be used in myriad ways. Serve it as a dip with chips, a garnish on Quick Black Bean Tostadas (page 218), a topping on Nachos (page 108), or an accompaniment to a baked potato.

2 medium tomatoes, cored and finely chopped (about 2 cups)

1 small onion, finely chopped (about 1 cup)

¼ cup finely chopped fresh cilantro

½ jalapeño pepper, seeded and finely chopped (about 2 tablespoons; optional)

In a medium bowl, stir together the tomatoes, onion, cilantro, and jalapeño (if using) until well combined. Chill in the refrigerator until ready to use.

Storage: Store in an airtight container in the refrigerator for 4 to 5 days.

Green Pea Guacamole

Makes about 3 cups ■ Ready in 10 minutes

This guacamole has great flavor and a lighter texture than guacamole made with avocado alone, plus it holds its lovely bright green color for longer. Serve with tortilla chips or with Nachos (page 108), Quick Black Bean Tostadas (page 218), Mexican Bowls (page 200), or Vegetable Breakfast Quesadillas (page 100).

2 cups frozen green peas, rinsed and drained

1 wedge from medium onion (about 1 inch wide)

4 small garlic cloves, minced (about 2 teaspoons)

1 jalapeño pepper, stemmed and seeded

1 Hass avocado, peeled, pitted, and mashed (about ¾ cup)

1 medium tomato, cut into ¼-inch dice (about 1 cup)

2 scallions, white and green parts, thinly sliced (about ½ cup)

2 tablespoons finely chopped fresh cilantro

2 tablespoons fresh lime juice (from 1 lime)

Sea salt and freshly ground black pepper

1. In a medium saucepan, bring 1½ cups water to a boil over medium-high heat. Add the green peas and cook until softened but not falling apart, about 5 minutes. Drain and run the peas under cold water to stop the cooking process.

2. Transfer the peas to a blender. Add the onion, garlic, and jalapeño and blend until smooth, adding a small amount of water as necessary to keep the mixture moving.

3. Transfer to a medium bowl. Add the mashed avocado, tomato, scallions, cilantro, lime juice, and salt and pepper to taste.

4. Cover the bowl and refrigerate until cold. Serve chilled.

Storage: Store in an airtight container in the refrigerator for 3 to 4 days.

RECIPES

Nacho Cheese

Makes about 4 cups ■ Ready in 35 minutes

This yummy "cheese" is great for making Nachos (page 108), to top cheesy casseroles, serve as a dip, or spread on tortillas to make cheese quesadillas. The weight of the prepared carrot is a little more important in this case than in other preparations, because it needs to be in good balance with the other ingredients for best flavor and color.

1 pound Yukon Gold potatoes (about 2 medium), peeled and cut into 1-inch pieces

5 ounces carrot (about 1 very large), peeled and cut into 1-inch pieces (about 1 cup)

2 cups unsweetened, unflavored plant milk

1 cup nutritional yeast

1 tablespoon fresh lemon juice (from ½ lemon)

1 tablespoon onion powder

Sea salt and freshly ground black pepper

1. Place a steamer basket in a sauté or saucepan, and add 1 to 2 inches of water to the pan. Cover and bring to a simmer. Place the potatoes and carrot in the steamer, cover, and steam until very tender when pierced with a fork, about 15 minutes.

2. Transfer to a blender and let cool until warm. Add the milk, nutritional yeast, lemon juice, onion powder, and salt and pepper to taste. Blend until you achieve a smooth, creamy, spreadable texture; add water if needed to reach the right consistency. Use at once or refrigerate until ready to use.

Storage: Store in an airtight container in the refrigerator for 4 to 5 days.

Yukon Golden Cheese

Makes about 3 cups ■ *Ready in 25 minutes*

This spreadable, pourable cheese sauce is good in baked dishes such as Vegetable and Cheese Enchiladas (page 172) and Baked Ziti (page 171), as well as in lasagna and on top of pizza.

2 medium Yukon Gold potatoes (about 1 pound), peeled and cut into roughly 1-inch pieces

1½ cups unsweetened, unflavored plant milk

½ cup nutritional yeast

Sea salt and freshly ground black pepper

1. Place a steamer basket in a sauté or saucepan and add 1 to 2 inches of water to the pan. Cover and bring to a simmer. Place the potatoes in the steamer, cover, and steam until very tender when pierced with a fork, 10 to 15 minutes.

2. Transfer the potatoes to a blender and let cool. Add the milk, nutritional yeast, and salt and pepper to taste. Blend on medium speed just until the mixture is smooth, creamy, and spreadable. Add water as necessary to achieve the right consistency. Refrigerate until ready to use.

Storage: Store in an airtight container in the refrigerator for 4 to 5 days.

RECIPES

Cashew Crumble

Makes about 1 cup ■ Ready in 15 minutes

*Sprinkle this crumble over the Mac 'n Cheese (page 184), as well as
on any pasta, pizza, salad, or casserole for a tasty cheesy flavor.*

1 cup ground cashews
2 tablespoons nutritional yeast
2 teaspoons mild white miso
2 teaspoons low-sodium
  tamari or soy sauce

1. In a medium bowl, place the cashews and nutritional yeast and use a fork to stir until combined.
2. In a small bowl, stir together the miso and tamari and pour the mixture over the cashews. Stir until well combined.
3. Let stand until the moisture is absorbed, about 10 minutes. Transfer to an airtight container and keep refrigerated until needed.

Storage: Store in an airtight container in the refrigerator for up to 10 days.

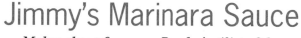

Jimmy's Marinara Sauce

Makes about 6 cups ■ *Ready in 1¾ to 2 hours*

On a summer trip to New York, my boyfriend and I had the opportunity to enjoy our friend Jimmy Hennessy's truly delicious marinara sauce over pasta. Jimmy says the secret to his sauce is using the variety of tomatoes grown in the San Marzano region of Italy. These large plum tomatoes can be found in many supermarkets and also online. Here is my version of his fantastic recipe. It doesn't take much active time on the cook's part and it stores beautifully.

4 heads of garlic

4 (14.5-ounce) cans crushed tomatoes, preferably San Marzano

¼ cup dried oregano

Sea salt and freshly ground black pepper

½ cup fresh basil, roughly chopped

1. Preheat the oven to 400°F.
2. Place the whole heads of garlic on a baking sheet and bake until soft to the touch, 40 to 45 minutes. Let cool.
3. Cut the narrow end off each garlic head and squeeze out the cloves into a small bowl. Mash the garlic into a paste.
4. Place the tomatoes, oregano, and mashed garlic in a large sauté pan. Bring to a simmer over medium heat and cook, stirring occasionally, until the sauce thickens, 45 minutes to an hour.
5. Add salt and pepper to taste and stir in the fresh basil. Serve hot over cooked pasta, or let cool and use for pizza topping.

Storage: Store in an airtight container in the refrigerator for up to 7 days or in the freezer for 2 to 3 months.

Cremini Mushroom Gravy

Makes about 4 cups ■ *Ready in 35 minutes*

*This gravy is an integral part of the Lentil Shepherd's Pie
(page 182). It's also satisfying served over cooked pasta, or you
can stir it into warm cooked rice to make a quick risotto.*

1 small onion, finely chopped
(about 1 cup)

3 small garlic cloves, minced
(about ½ tablespoon)

1 pound cremini mushrooms,
trimmed and sliced (about
6 cups)

½ tablespoon dried thyme, or
1 tablespoon fresh thyme
leaves

½ tablespoon dried sage, or
1 tablespoon chopped fresh
sage leaves

Sea salt and freshly ground
black pepper

3 tablespoons oat flour

3 cups Vegetable Stock
(page 262) or no-oil,
low-sodium store-bought or
water, plus more as needed

1 tablespoon white wine
vinegar

1. Place the onion and garlic in a saucepan with
   ½ cup water. Cook, covered, over medium-low heat
   until the onion is translucent, 5 to 10 minutes.

2. Add the mushrooms, thyme, sage, and salt
   and pepper to taste, and increase the heat to
   medium. Cook, uncovered, until the mushrooms
   are completely cooked, stirring occasionally,
   about 10 minutes.

3. Meanwhile, in a medium bowl, mix the flour
   with the vegetable stock and vinegar and whisk
   until smooth.

4. Stirring constantly, slowly add the slurry to
   the mushrooms. Bring the gravy to a boil, then
   reduce the heat and simmer until thickened,
   about 5 minutes. If the mixture is too thick, add
   some vegetable stock or water to thin it.

5. Remove from the heat and let cool. Pour
   half the gravy into a blender and blend
   until smooth. Return the blended portion
   to the saucepan with the remaining gravy.
   (Alternatively, blend all of the gravy until
   smooth.) Set aside until needed.

Storage: Store in an airtight container in the refrigerator for
4 to 5 days. Reheat in a medium saucepan over low heat just
before serving.

Tomato Ketchup

Makes about 3 cups ■ Ready in 2½ hours

So much of store-bought ketchup is high in sugar and salt. Stored in sterilized jars, this fresher version will keep for several months.

2 pounds ripe tomatoes, cut into 1-inch dice (about 5 cups)

1 small red onion, finely chopped (about 1 cup)

6 to 8 dates, pitted

1½ cups Vegetable Stock (page 262) or no-oil, low-sodium store-bought

¼ cup apple cider vinegar

¼ cup no-salt-added tomato paste

½ tablespoon ground pasilla chile

½ tablespoon ground New Mexico chile

¼ teaspoon freshly ground black pepper

Pinch of sea salt

1. In a large saucepan, place the tomatoes, onion, dates, and vegetable stock. Bring to a boil over medium heat, then reduce the heat and simmer until the vegetables are cooked completely, about 30 minutes. Remove from the heat and let cool for a few minutes.

2. Transfer the tomato mixture to a blender. Add 1 cup water, the vinegar, tomato paste, ground chiles, pepper, and salt, and blend until smooth.

3. Rinse out the saucepan and return the mixture to the pan. Simmer, stirring occasionally, over medium heat until the mixture cooks down to a thick paste, 1 to 1½ hours.

4. Meanwhile, have ready about three 8-ounce mason jars and lids. Bring a large pot of water to a boil. Place the jars and lids in the water, making sure they are completely submerged, and boil for 10 minutes. Use tongs to remove the jars and lids from the water and transfer to a cooling rack or towel to dry. (Alternatively, use about two 12-ounce sauce bottles; there is no need to sterilize the bottle caps.)

5. Pour the hot ketchup into the sterilized jars and close tightly. Let cool completely.

Storage: Store in the refrigerator; unopened jars will keep for 6 to 8 months and opened jars will keep for 1 month.

RECIPES

Barbecue Sauce

Makes about 5 cups ■ *Ready in 30 minutes*

This sauce is neither too sweet nor too spicy, and it goes well with any grain or roasted seasonal vegetables. The optional chipotle chile adds a smoky heat.

1 cup Date Paste (page 265)
¼ cup white wine vinegar
¼ cup oat flour
2 tablespoons no-salt-added tomato paste
2 tablespoons garlic powder
2 tablespoons onion powder
2 tablespoons smoked paprika
1½ tablespoons vegan Worcestershire sauce
1½ tablespoons low-sodium tamari or soy sauce
2 teaspoons prepared yellow mustard
2 (1-inch) pieces canned chipotle chile in adobo sauce, or to taste (optional)

1. In a blender, place 4 cups water, the date paste, vinegar, oat flour, tomato paste, garlic powder, onion powder, smoked paprika, Worcestershire sauce, tamari, mustard, and chipotle (if using). Blend until smooth.

2. Transfer the mixture to a saucepan and cook over medium heat, stirring occasionally, until the sauce thickens and the flavors have blended, 15 to 20 minutes. Use at once or store until needed.

Storage: Store in an airtight container in the refrigerator for up to 10 days.

Cilantro Lime Chutney

Makes about 2½ cups ■ Ready in 10 minutes

This is a variation on traditional Indian cilantro chutney. The green peas and sesame seed paste (tahini) give it a rich texture.

2 cups frozen green peas

4 cups cilantro leaves and tender stems (from about 1 bunch)

2 tablespoons sesame seed paste (tahini)

1 jalapeño pepper, stemmed and seeded (optional)

¼ cup fresh lime juice (from 2 limes)

1 teaspoon cumin seeds

½ tablespoon Date Paste (page 265)

1 small garlic clove, coarsely chopped (about ½ teaspoon)

Sea salt

1. Bring 1½ cups water to a boil over medium-high heat in a small saucepan. Add the green peas and cook until soft, 8 to 10 minutes. Drain and rinse with cold water.

2. Transfer the peas to a blender. Add 1 cup water and the cilantro, sesame seed paste, jalapeño (if using), lime juice, cumin seeds, date paste, garlic, and salt to taste. Blend until creamy.

3. Transfer to an airtight container and chill in the refrigerator for 1 hour before serving.

Storage: Store in the refrigerator for 4 to 5 days.

RECIPES

Tomatillo Sauce

Makes about 4 cups ■ *Ready in 35 minutes*

This tomatillo sauce can be served as a salsa with tortilla chips or as a sauce over steamed grains or vegetables, as it is in the Tomatillo Sauce over Potatoes (page 215). Mexican oregano gives the dish an authentic flavor. You can find it in Mexican markets. You can certainly use Mediterranean oregano instead.

1 pound tomatillos (10 to 12), husks removed, rinsed well

½ medium onion, halved

2 jalapeño peppers, stemmed and seeded (optional)

3 small garlic cloves

½ bunch fresh cilantro (1 cup packed leaves and tender stems), plus more for garnish

1 teaspoon dried Mexican oregano

¼ teaspoon ground cumin

Sea salt

1. Place the tomatillos, onion, jalapeños (if using), garlic, and 2 cups water in a large saucepan. Cover and cook over medium heat for 20 minutes. Remove from the heat, uncover, and let cool for about 10 minutes.

2. Transfer the tomatillo mixture to a blender. Add the cilantro, oregano, cumin, and salt to taste. Blend into a smooth sauce. Use at once or refrigerate until ready to use.

Store: Store in an airtight container in the refrigerator for 5 to 7 days.

Tahini Sauce

Makes about 1½ cups ■ *Ready in 10 minutes (plus 30 minutes for chilling)*

This basic tahini sauce is very pleasing to kids. If you want to add a little zing, stir in ¼ cup chopped fresh tarragon or chives. Serve this sauce with Falafel Sandwiches (page 128), Couscous Bowls (page 199), Samosa Stuffed Muffins (page 210), and Cornbread (page 214), or as a dipping sauce for fresh vegetables.

½ cup sesame seed paste (tahini)

¼ cup fresh lemon juice (from 2 lemons)

3 small garlic cloves, minced (about ½ tablespoon)

Sea salt and freshly ground black pepper

Place the sesame seed paste, lemon juice, garlic, salt and pepper to taste, and 1 cup water in a blender. Blend to a smooth, pourable consistency. If the sauce is too thick, add water 1 tablespoon at a time to loosen it. Store in the refrigerator for at least 30 minutes before serving.

Storage: Store in an airtight container in the refrigerator for up to 7 days.

Ranch Dressing

Makes about 2 cups ■ Ready in 10 minutes

This nice alternative to store-bought oily ranch dressing comes together quickly. Fresh herbs give it authentic flavor, but you can certainly use dried herbs in their place. Serve over lightly steamed or raw vegetables, use as a salad dressing, or serve with Marinated Tempeh (page 217).

1 (12-ounce) package soft silken tofu (see Note)

1½ teaspoons white wine vinegar

2 teaspoons onion powder

1½ teaspoons garlic powder

Sea salt and freshly ground black pepper

2 teaspoons chopped fresh parsley, or ½ teaspoon dried

2 teaspoons chopped fresh dill, or ½ teaspoon dried

2 teaspoons chopped fresh chives, or ½ teaspoon dried

1. In a blender, place the tofu, vinegar, onion powder, garlic powder, and salt and pepper to taste. Blend until creamy.
2. Transfer to a medium bowl and stir in the parsley, dill, and chives. Mix well and adjust the seasoning. Chill before serving.

Storage: Store in an airtight container in the refrigerator for 3 to 4 days.

Note: Alternatively, use 1 (15-ounce) can rinsed and drained white beans (about 1½ cups) and ½ cup unsweetened, unflavored plant milk in place of the tofu.

RECIPES

Thousand Island Dressing

Makes about 2 cups ■ *Ready in 15 minutes*

This dressing has all the bright, tangy-sweet flavor of classic Thousand Island, but without the heavy mayonnaise. Serve it as a sandwich spread and/or salad dressing. It can be a dipping sauce with crudités or pita chips or it can be spread on whole-grain toast piled with lettuce, tomatoes, and thinly sliced onion.

1 (15-ounce) can white beans, rinsed and drained (about 1½ cups)

1 cup unsweetened, unflavored plant milk

3 tablespoons Tomato Ketchup (page 237) or store-bought

1 teaspoon Dijon mustard

1 teaspoon white wine vinegar

1 small garlic clove

¼ teaspoon hot sauce (optional)

Sea salt and freshly ground black pepper

2 tablespoons finely chopped hearts of palm

2 tablespoons low-sodium sweet pickle relish or finely chopped sweet pickle (optional)

1 tablespoon finely diced onion or shallot

1 tablespoon finely diced red bell pepper

1 teaspoon dried parsley, or ½ tablespoon finely chopped fresh

1. In a blender, place the beans, milk, ketchup, mustard, vinegar, garlic, hot sauce (if using), and salt and pepper to taste. Blend until smooth and creamy.

2. Transfer to a medium bowl and stir in the hearts of palm, relish (if using), onion, bell pepper, and parsley. Taste and adjust the seasoning. Refrigerate until ready to use.

Storage: Store in an airtight container in the refrigerator for 3 to 4 days.

RECIPES

RECIPES

Carrot, Orange, and Ginger Dressing

Makes about 2 cups ■ *Ready in 25 minutes*

This dressing has a very refreshing ginger-orange taste that goes well with a mixed greens and grains salad. Both orange zest and segments are used here, but they are added at different times, so be sure to grate the orange zest before peeling and cutting the orange.

1 large carrot, cut into ½-inch coins (about 1 cup)

1 teaspoon grated fresh ginger

½ medium orange, peeled and sectioned, cut into 1-inch pieces (about ½ cup)

¼ cup fresh lemon juice (from 2 lemons)

½ tablespoon white wine vinegar

1 small garlic clove

1 tablespoon pure maple syrup (optional)

1 tablespoon grated orange zest

Sea salt and freshly ground black pepper

2 tablespoons finely chopped fresh parsley

1. Place the carrot, ginger, and ½ cup water in a small saucepan. Cover and cook over medium heat until the carrot is tender, about 10 minutes.

2. Add the orange pieces and cook, covered, until the orange is lightly cooked, about 5 minutes. Remove the pan from the heat and let the mixture cool.

3. Transfer the orange mixture to a blender and add ½ cup water along with the lemon juice, vinegar, garlic, maple syrup (if using), orange zest, and salt and pepper to taste. Blend until smooth.

4. Add the parsley and pulse a few times to mix well. Transfer to an airtight container and chill until ready to serve.

Storage: Store in the refrigerator for 4 to 5 days.

Miso Lime Dressing

Makes about 2 cups ■ *Ready in 10 minutes*

This dressing goes well with the Tokyo Bowls (page 202) or any salad greens or in a salad of chopped seasonal vegetables.

½ cup fresh lime juice
(from 2 limes)

¼ cup mild white miso

2 tablespoons sesame seed
paste (tahini)

4 to 6 small garlic cloves

1½ tablespoons grated ginger

1½ tablespoons Date Paste
(page 265)

1 teaspoon minced fresh
parsley, or ½ teaspoon dried

Sea salt and freshly ground
black pepper

1. In a blender, place 1 cup water, the lime juice, miso, sesame seed paste, garlic, ginger, date paste, parsley, and salt and pepper to taste. Blend until smooth.

2. Transfer to a jar with a tight-fitting lid and refrigerate until cold before using.

Storage: Store in the refrigerator for up to 1 week.

DESSERTS

Fudgy Brownies

Makes 24 (1½-inch) squares ■ *Ready in 50 minutes*

You can't go wrong with these fudgy brownies. They are always a big hit with a crowd. Black beans give the brownies their moist texture, and the beans' neutral flavor works well with the chocolate. Using a relatively small amount of flour prevents the brownies from getting too heavy.

¾ cup natural unsweetened cocoa powder

⅓ cup oat flour

⅓ cup sorghum flour

¼ cup almond flour

1 teaspoon baking powder

Pinch of sea salt

1 (15-ounce) can black beans, rinsed and drained (about 1½ cups)

1 cup Date Paste (page 265)

½ cup unsweetened applesauce

½ cup unsweetened, unflavored plant milk

2 tablespoons pure maple syrup

1 teaspoon pure vanilla extract

¼ cup vegan chocolate chips

½ cup chopped walnuts (optional)

1. Preheat the oven to 350°F. Line the bottom and sides of a 9 × 13-inch baking dish with parchment paper.

2. In a large bowl, whisk together the cocoa powder, oat flour, sorghum flour, almond flour, baking powder, and salt. Set aside.

3. In a food processor, place the beans, date paste, applesauce, milk, maple syrup, and vanilla. Process until smooth.

4. Pour the liquid mixture into the dry ingredients. Stir until well blended.

5. Stir in the chocolate chips and half of the walnuts (if using). Transfer the batter to the prepared baking pan. Sprinkle with the remaining walnuts (if using).

6. Bake until the top is dry and firm, about 40 minutes. Cool in the pan on a rack. Slice into 24 squares.

Storage: Store in an airtight container in the refrigerator for 3 to 4 days.

Crunchy Grain, Seed, and Dried Fruit Bars

Makes 20 (2 × 2-inch) bars ■ *Ready in 2½ hours*

These bars take a little while to bake and completely cool, but the relatively short active time and an ingredient list primarily composed of pantry staples more than make up for that. Plus, the end result is delicious, and always a hit with both kids and grown-ups. They taste better the day after baking and store very well.

1 tablespoon dry millet, rinsed and drained

1 tablespoon dry quinoa, rinsed and drained

2 cups old-fashioned rolled oats

½ cup unsalted pumpkin seeds

½ cup unsalted sunflower seeds

1 cup Date Paste (page 265)

½ cup unsweetened applesauce

½ cup finely chopped dried figs

¼ cup finely chopped dried apricots

¼ cup raisins

2 tablespoons grated orange zest

1. Preheat the oven to 200°F. Line a baking sheet with parchment paper.

2. In a large skillet, toast the millet and quinoa over medium heat, stirring occasionally, until completely dry and toasty, 5 to 7 minutes.

3. Add the oats, pumpkin seeds, and sunflower seeds to the skillet and toast until the seeds are toasted lightly brown, about 10 minutes.

4. Transfer the toasted grains and seeds to a large bowl. Add the date paste, applesauce, figs, apricots, raisins, and orange zest and mix well.

5. Use your hands to spread the mixture on the prepared baking sheet into an evenly thick, roughly 8 x 10-inch rectangle.

6. Bake until firm and crisp on top, about 2 hours. Let cool completely in the pan. Cut into 20 squares.

Storage: Store in an airtight container at room temperature for up to 1 week.

RECIPES

Apple-Cinnamon Cookies

Makes 20 to 24 (3-inch) cookies ■ *Ready in 50 minutes*

These gluten-free cookies have a crisp outside and a nice, soft inside with a little crunch from the cornmeal. Their flavor is reminiscent of gingerbread. If gluten is not a concern, you can replace the sorghum and oat flours with whole wheat or spelt flour.

1½ cups coarse cornmeal

¾ cup gluten-free oat flour

¾ cup sorghum flour

1 teaspoon ground cinnamon

2 pinches of ground cloves

1 teaspoon baking soda

Pinch of sea salt

1 cup unsweetened applesauce

1 cup pure maple syrup

1 cup unsalted natural almond or sesame butter

2 tablespoons ground flaxseed

½ cup unsweetened dried apple, finely chopped (see Note)

½ cup slivered or sliced almonds

1. Arrange two baking racks in the upper and lower thirds of the oven. Preheat the oven to 350°F. Line two baking sheets with parchment paper.

2. In a large bowl, whisk together the cornmeal, oat flour, sorghum flour, cinnamon, cloves, baking soda, and salt until well blended.

3. In a medium bowl, whisk together the applesauce, maple syrup, almond butter, and ground flaxseed until well blended.

4. Add the liquid ingredients and the dried apple to the dry mixture. Use a wooden spoon to mix gently but well.

5. Drop 1½ to 2 tablespoons of dough for each cookie onto the prepared baking sheets, spacing about 1½ inches apart. Flatten each with the back of a spoon and sprinkle with the slivered almonds.

6. Bake until the tops are lightly browned, about 35 minutes (after about 20 minutes, rotate the pans from lower to upper racks and back to front for even baking).

7. Cool on the baking sheets for 5 minutes. Remove to wire racks. Cool completely.

Storage: Store in an airtight container at room temperature for up to 4 days or in the freezer for up to 1 month.

Note: Be sure to use soft, dried apples, not crisp, freeze-dried apples.

RECIPES

RECIPES

Fruity Cupcakes with Orange Frosting

Makes 12 cupcakes ■ Ready in 1¼ hours

Sweet potatoes are a great base for frosting for many reasons. The flesh lends creaminess without any added nuts or other fats; they are naturally sweet, so you don't need much added sweetener; and the natural flavor is a great neutral base on which to build the orange flavor with orange juice and zest.

FOR THE CUPCAKES

2 cups buckwheat or oat flour

¼ cup almond flour

1¼ teaspoons baking powder

1 teaspoon baking soda

Pinch of sea salt

8 ounces fresh or frozen mango or pineapple, cut into 1-inch cubes (about 1¾ cups)

1 cup unsweetened, unflavored plant milk

¾ cup Date Paste (page 265)

2 tablespoons pure maple syrup

2 tablespoons sesame seed paste (tahini)

1 teaspoon pure vanilla extract

1 teaspoon apple cider vinegar

FOR THE FROSTING

1 pound regular or white-fleshed sweet potatoes (about 2 medium), peeled and cut into 1-inch pieces (about 4 cups)

1 medium carrot, peeled and cut into ¼-inch dice (about ½ cup)

1. Preheat the oven to 350°F. Line a standard cupcake pan with cupcake liners.

2. Make the cupcakes: In a large bowl, whisk together the flours, baking powder, baking soda, and salt until well blended. Set aside.

3. In a blender, place the mango, milk, date paste, maple syrup, sesame seed paste, vanilla, and vinegar. Blend until smooth.

4. Pour the liquid ingredients over the dry mixture and stir just until the flour is incorporated and the batter is smooth. (Rinse the blender; you'll need it for the frosting.)

5. Divide the batter among the lined cups. Bake until a toothpick inserted into the center of a cupcake comes out clean, 30 to 40 minutes.

6. Let the cupcakes cool in the pan for a few minutes, then transfer them to a rack to cool completely.

7. Make the frosting: Place a steamer basket into a sauté or saucepan, and add 1 to 2 inches of water to the pan. Cover and bring to a simmer. Place the sweet potatoes and carrot in the steamer, cover, and steam until very tender

¼ to ½ cup fresh orange juice

1 teaspoon grated orange zest

¼ cup pure maple syrup, or
  as needed (optional)

½ cup raspberries or other
  fresh berries, for garnish

when pierced with a fork, about 15 minutes.
Transfer to a large bowl to cool.

8. In the blender, place the sweet potatoes and
   carrot, ¼ cup of the orange juice, and the zest.
   Blend until smooth and creamy, adding as much
   of the remaining orange juice as necessary to
   keep the mixture moving. Add the maple syrup
   to taste if the frosting is not sweet enough or
   as needed to keep the mixture from sticking to
   the blender. (If not using immediately, store in
   an airtight container in the refrigerator until
   needed.)

9. Frost the cooled cupcakes and decorate each
   with 1 or 2 raspberries.

Storage: Store in an airtight container in the refrigerator until
ready to serve or for 3 to 4 days.

Layer Cake with Vanilla Frosting 📷

Makes 1 (9-inch) cake ■ *Ready in 2 hours*

This is a tasty and very pretty cake, perfect for birthday celebrations. It takes a bit of time and labor to prepare, but it's very much worth it, as it's a real crowd-pleaser—for kids and adults alike. Try to have them figure out what makes the frosting so creamy; most will never guess that the secret is white beans. If you have a small blender, like the ones that often come as attachments with stick blenders, it's very useful for making the frosting.

FOR THE CAKE

¾ cup unsweetened, unflavored plant milk

1 tablespoon apple cider vinegar

1 tablespoon ground flaxseed

¾ cup pure maple syrup

2 teaspoons pure vanilla extract

1¾ cups whole wheat pastry flour

½ cup almond flour

1 teaspoon grated nutmeg

1 teaspoon ground cinnamon

1 teaspoon baking powder

1 teaspoon baking soda

¼ teaspoon sea salt

FOR THE FROSTING AND FILLING

1 (15-ounce) can white beans, rinsed and drained (about 1½ cups)

½ cup pure maple syrup

⅓ cup almond flour

2 teaspoons pure vanilla extract

1. Preheat the oven to 350°F. Line the bottom of a 9-inch springform cake pan with a round piece of parchment paper.

2. Make the cake: In a medium bowl, whisk together the milk, vinegar, and ground flaxseed. Let stand for 10 minutes.

3. Whisk in the maple syrup and vanilla. Set aside.

4. In a large bowl, whisk together the flours, nutmeg, cinnamon, baking powder, baking soda, and salt until well blended.

5. Add the liquid ingredients to the dry mixture and use a wooden spoon or spatula to mix well.

6. Pour the batter into the prepared cake pan. Bake until a toothpick inserted in the middle of the cake comes out dry, 45 to 50 minutes.

7. Cool the cake in the pan for 10 minutes. Remove the sides of the pan. Invert onto a cooling rack and remove the parchment paper

from the bottom. Flip the cake upright and let cool completely.

8. Make the frosting: In a medium saucepan, place the beans, maple syrup, almond flour, vanilla, and cinnamon. Cook over medium-low heat for about 5 minutes so that the flavors can merge. Remove from the heat and let cool for about 10 minutes.

9. Transfer to a blender and blend until smooth and spreadable; add a very small amount of water only if absolutely needed to keep the mixture moving in the blender.

10. Transfer to a bowl and refrigerate for at least 1 hour before using.

Pinch of ground cinnamon
½ cup fruit-sweetened jam
1 to 1½ cups fresh mixed berries, for garnish

11. Assemble the cake: Run a large knife under water (to prevent sticking), then cut the cake horizontally into two equal layers.

12. Place the bottom cake layer cut side up on a cake plate. Spread the jam evenly on the layer, smoothing it across almost the entire surface, but leaving about ½ inch around the outside untouched (so that the jam does not seep out when the top layer is added).

13. Place the top cake layer on the jam. Cover the top and sides of the cake with the frosting.

14. Chill the cake for at least 1 hour before serving. If making the cake more than a few hours in advance, decorate with the berries just before serving.

Storage: Store in the refrigerator for up to 4 days.

254

FORKS OVER KNIVES FAMILY

Chocolate Pie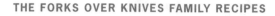

Makes 1 (9-inch) pie ■ *Ready in 1½ hours (plus at least 1 hour for chilling)*

*Fresh acorn squash makes a creamy and smooth chocolate
filling. To save time you can use canned pumpkin instead; the
filling won't be as smooth, but it will still taste delicious.*

FOR THE CRUST

1¼ cups old-fashioned rolled
  oats

¾ cup cashews

¾ cup sorghum flour, plus
  more as needed

Pinch of sea salt

½ cup pure maple syrup

1 teaspoon pure vanilla
  extract

FOR THE FILLING

6 cups peeled and cubed
  acorn squash in 1-inch
  pieces (about 1¾ pounds),
  or 2 (15-ounce) cans
  pumpkin

1½ cups Date Paste
  (page 265)

¼ cup unsweetened,
  unflavored plant milk

¾ cup natural unsweetened
  cocoa powder

1½ teaspoons pure vanilla
  extract

¼ cup chopped pecans,
  for garnish

1. Preheat the oven to 350°F. Line the base of a
   9-inch pie plate with parchment paper.

2. Make the crust: In a food processor, place the
   oats, cashews, flour, and salt and grind to a fine
   meal. Add the maple syrup and vanilla extract
   and pulse until the mixture starts to bind
   together.

3. Transfer about half the mixture to the prepared
   pie dish and pat it into an even, thin crust on
   the bottom of the dish. If the mixture is too
   sticky to handle, wet your fingers with some
   water or use a little sorghum flour. Press the
   remaining crust mixture evenly up the sides of
   the pan and form a nice edge around the top
   rim of the pie plate. Prick the dough with a
   fork in a few places (to prevent puffing during
   baking).

4. Bake the crust until lightly brown and crisp,
   20 to 30 minutes. Let cool completely.

5. Make the filling: If using fresh squash, place a
   steamer basket into a sauté or saucepan, and
   add 1 to 2 inches of water to the pan. Cover
   and bring to a simmer. Place the squash in the

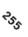

steamer, cover, and steam until very tender when pierced with a fork, about 15 minutes. Transfer the squash to a bowl to cool completely.

6. Transfer the squash or canned pumpkin (if using) to a food processor and add the date paste, milk, cocoa powder, and vanilla. Blend until smooth.

7. Scrape the chocolate filling into the crust and spread evenly. Chill in the refrigerator for at least 1 hour. Decorate with the pecans before serving.

Spiced Chocolate Pie

For a chocolate twist on the traditional Thanksgiving pumpkin pie, omit the vanilla in the filling and add instead ½ teaspoon ground cinnamon, ¼ teaspoon ground allspice, and ¼ teaspoon grated nutmeg.

RECIPES

Peanut Butter Ice "Cream"

Makes about 1 quart ■ Ready in 1 hour (plus 5 to 6 hours for freezing)

It can be hard to get all the good flavor of peanut butter into ice cream without it being very heavy. But this one succeeds, thanks to the almond milk. A generous amount of vanilla underscores and enhances the great flavor. Serve this by itself or in a sundae (see page 257).

2 cups Almond Milk (page 264) or unsweetened, unflavored store-bought

½ cup pure maple syrup

¼ cup unsalted natural smooth peanut butter

2 teaspoons pure vanilla extract

4 medium bananas, peeled, cut into thick slices, and frozen

1. Have ready two mini cupcake pans or two to three ice cube trays.
2. In a small saucepan, bring the almond milk and maple syrup to a simmer. Simmer for 10 to 15 minutes, until the milk thickens slightly. Remove from the heat and let cool.
3. Transfer the cooled almond milk to a blender. Add the peanut butter and vanilla, and blend until smooth.
4. Pour the mixture into the mini cupcake pans or ice cube trays. Freeze for 5 to 6 hours or until hard.
5. Place the frozen peanut butter mixture into a blender. Add the frozen bananas. Blend into a creamy ice-cream-like texture. If the blade isn't turning well, turn off the blender and let the mixture stand for a few minutes to soften slightly.
6. Transfer the ice "cream" to a container with a lid. Cover and freeze until ready to serve.

Storage: Store in the freezer for up to 15 days.

Chocolate Sundae with Caramelized Bananas

Makes about 6 sundaes, with about 1¾ cups chocolate sauce ■ *Ready in 20 minutes*

Chocolate sundaes are the quintessential childhood treat, and this one—which combines peanut butter ice cream, caramelized bananas, roasted almonds, and chocolate sauce—is downright heavenly. If the Peanut Butter Ice "Cream" isn't made already or you don't have time to make it, you can create a quickie ice cream instead by blending almost any frozen fruit with frozen bananas.

FOR THE CHOCOLATE SAUCE

1 cup unsweetened applesauce

⅓ cup unsweetened, unflavored plant milk

½ cup Date Paste (page 265), or ¼ cup pure maple syrup

2 tablespoons natural unsweetened cocoa powder

1 tablespoon sesame seed paste (tahini)

½ tablespoon pure vanilla extract

FOR THE SUNDAES

3 ripe medium bananas, peeled

1 quart Peanut Butter Ice "Cream" (page 256)

2 tablespoons chopped roasted almonds

1. Make the chocolate sauce: In a blender, place the applesauce, milk, date paste, cocoa powder, sesame seed paste, and vanilla. Blend until creamy, scraping down the sides of the blender once or twice.

2. Transfer to a jar or squeeze bottle with a lid, and chill in the refrigerator until ready to serve.

3. Make the sundaes: Heat a medium nonstick skillet over medium heat. Cook the bananas until lightly browned in spots, about 5 minutes. Flip the bananas and continue to cook until lightly browned on the other side, about 5 minutes. Remove from the heat and cut the bananas into 1-inch pieces.

4. For each sundae, place 2 scoops of ice cream in a sundae bowl. Top with a few pieces of caramelized bananas. Drizzle the chocolate sauce over, and sprinkle some chopped almonds on top. Serve at once.

Storage: Store in an airtight container in the refrigerator for 5 to 7 days.

RECIPES

Tricolor Ice "Creamcakes"

Makes 6 to 9 cupcakes ■ *Ready in 1 hour (plus about 6 hours for freezing)*

Here's a fun and festive way to serve fruit ice cream: layer three different kinds in cupcake liners and call them ice creamcakes! Kept covered in the freezer, the creamcakes can be stored for weeks, making it well worth the effort to prepare a big batch to have on hand. If you need to use the cupcake tray in the meantime, you can unmold and store the creamcakes in a separate container, as instructed on page 259. This is a very pretty and tasty combination for tricolor creamcakes, but naturally you can use whatever combination you like.

2 cups frozen mixed berries
2 medium bananas, cut into 2 or 3 pieces and frozen
2 cups frozen diced mango

1. Have ready one or two silicone cupcake pans (see Note) and two baking sheets.
2. Place the berries in a blender, and blend until smooth; work quickly so that the berries don't defrost. Fill each of 6 to 9 cupcake cups about ⅓ full, dividing the berries evenly among the cups.
3. Place the cupcake pan on a baking sheet and store in the freezer.
4. Rinse the blender thoroughly and blend the frozen bananas until creamy.
5. Remove the cupcake pan and baking sheet from the freezer. Divide the banana puree evenly among the cups of berries. Return to the freezer.
6. Place the frozen mango in the blender (there's no need to rinse the blender unless desired). Blend until creamy and smooth.

7. Remove the cupcake pan from the freezer. Divide the frozen mango evenly among the cups.

8. Cover the cupcake pan with the remaining baking sheet or with plastic wrap. Freeze until set, at least 6 hours.

9. Unmold when ready to serve.

Storage: Unmold the frozen creamcakes and store in an airtight container in the freezer for 2 to 3 weeks.

Note: The volume of each individual cup in standard silicone cupcake pans can vary and is generally between ⅓ and ½ cup. If your pan has the larger cups, you'll get about 6 creamcakes; if it has the smaller cups, the recipe will yield about 9.

Orange 'n Berry Ice Pops 📷

Makes 8 ice pops ■ *Ready in 1¼ hours (plus about 6 hours for freezing)*

*Kids love these colorful orange ice pops with their pink-and-purple tips
and sweet and tangy flavor. They are the quintessential summertime treat.
If you don't have ice pop molds, use small paper cups and wooden ice pop
sticks. When ready to serve, just peel the cups away from the ice pops.*

1¼ cups unsweetened pineapple or apple juice

1 tablespoon arrowroot powder

¼ cup pure maple syrup

2 tablespoons fresh lemon juice

½ cup frozen or fresh berries, pulsed in a blender until crushed

1½ cups fresh orange juice

1 orange, peeled and cut into ½-inch pieces (about 1 cup)

1. Have ready eight 3-ounce ice pop molds or eight paper cups and wooden sticks.

2. In a small bowl, mix ¼ cup of the pineapple juice with the arrowroot flour and set the slurry aside.

3. Pour the remaining 1 cup pineapple juice and the maple syrup into a small saucepan. Bring to a boil over medium heat, then reduce the heat to bring the juice to a simmer. Stirring constantly to prevent lumps from forming, add the slurry to the juice.

4. Add the lemon juice and mix well.

5. Transfer half the thickened pineapple juice (about ¾ cup) to a medium bowl. Add the berries to the bowl and stir well. Pour 1 to 2 tablespoons of the pineapple juice–berry mixture into each of the ice pop molds. Cover with plastic wrap and place in the freezer until frozen on the surface, about 1 hour.

6. Meanwhile, add the orange juice to the remaining thickened pineapple juice in the pan and stir until well blended. Set aside to cool.

7. Pour the orange juice mixture on top of the berries in the molds. Drop a few orange pieces into each mold. Put the stick and lid in place. (If using paper cups, tightly cover each with a piece of plastic wrap. Poke a hole through the center of the plastic and insert a wooden stick; the wrap will hold the stick in place.)
8. Freeze until solid, about 6 hours.
9. Unmold and serve.

Storage: Store the ice pops in the molds in the freezer for up to 3 weeks.

BASICS

Vegetable Stock

Makes about 14 cups ■ *Ready in 1 hour 40 minutes*

Sure, you can buy vegetable stock at the store, but making it at home is more economical and the end result pretty much always tastes far better than anything you can buy. Plus, it's the best way I know to use up all the vegetable scraps that are produced during cooking, like mushroom stems, herb stems, celery leaves, fennel fronds, and tomato seeds and skins. (Note that there are a few things that aren't great for stock: cauliflower, broccoli, cabbage, Brussels sprouts, bell peppers, beets, and greens, especially spinach.) I keep all usable scraps in a resealable bag in the freezer, and when the bag is full, I know it's time to make some stock. The stock itself stores beautifully in the fridge or freezer. The ingredients here are given as examples of vegetable scraps; use what you have on hand.

6 medium carrots

1 celery head

8 ounces cremini or button mushrooms

Any other leftover vegetable scraps

6 medium onions, peeled

1 garlic head

2 thyme sprigs

½ bunch fresh parsley

2 dried bay leaves

4 quarts water

1. Rinse the carrots, celery, mushrooms, and any other vegetable scraps you might be using; be sure to remove all the dirt and cut off any damaged or spoiled parts. Cut the vegetables into big pieces all about the same size, and place in a large stockpot.

2. Cut the onions into big pieces. Separate the garlic head into individual cloves; there is no need to peel them. Add the onions and garlic to the stockpot.

3. Place the thyme, parsley, and bay leaves in the stockpot and add the water. Bring to a boil over medium-high heat. Reduce the heat to low and

simmer, partially covered, for 45 to 60 minutes. Taste a piece of vegetable; if it still has its flavor, then the stock is not ready yet. Cook for another 30 minutes.

4. Immediately strain the stock through a fine-mesh sieve (or line a medium-mesh sieve with two or three layers of cheesecloth) into another pot or large bowl. Let cool completely.

Storage: Pour the stock into smaller airtight containers (about 4 cups each) with tight-fitting lids. I especially like mason jars for this because their shape makes them good space savers. Store for 2 to 3 days in the refrigerator or freeze for up to 2 months.

RECIPES

Almond Milk

Makes about 5 cups ■ *Ready in 10 minutes*

Most homemade almond milk is derived from blanched whole almonds, but the process can take more time than many busy families have to spare. This easy method—based on almond flour, which is simply ground almonds— gives you unsweetened, unflavored almond milk in just a few minutes.

1 cup almond flour

1. Place the almond flour in a blender with 4½ cups water. Blend until very creamy, 1 to 2 minutes.
2. Strain through a fine-mesh strainer into a bowl or other container.

Storage: Transfer the milk to a clean jar or bottle with a tight-fitting lid. Store in the refrigerator for 5 to 7 days.

Date Paste

Makes about 3 cups ■ Ready in 15 minutes (plus 3 to 8 hours for soaking)

If you use dates as the main sweetener in your cooking, it saves a lot of time to have them ready as a paste. Keep half the batch in the fridge and freeze the other half in a mason jar so you will always have some ready to go. Soak the dates overnight so that the blending process is easy. For best results, soak the dates in a flat-bottomed container so that they are all submerged in the water. The longer you soak them, the more quickly the dates will break down when blended.

**1 pound pitted dates
(about 4 cups)
1½ cups boiling water**

1. Place the dates in a wide, flat-bottomed container such as a saucepan and add the water (the dates should be partially to completely submerged). Cover the container and soak for at least 3 hours and up to 8 hours.
2. Transfer the dates and the soaking water to a food processor and blend into a smooth paste.

Storage: Transfer the paste to a jar with a tight-fitting lid. Store in the refrigerator for up to 1 month or in the freezer for 4 to 5 months.

Cornmeal Pizza Crust

Enough for 1 (9 × 13-inch) pizza or 6 (5-inch) mini pizzas ■ *Ready in 25 minutes*

This cornmeal crust is crispy, crunchy, and light. It's a great pizza crust, and it makes a delicious base for chili as well. To ensure that it is completely gluten-free, use gluten-free oat flour.

¾ cup fine cornmeal, plus more for dusting the pan

⅓ cup almond flour

1 cup oat flour

1 tablespoon ground flaxseed

1 teaspoon baking powder

½ teaspoon sea salt

¼ teaspoon ground cumin (optional)

¾ cup unsweetened, unflavored plant milk, lukewarm, plus more to brush the crust

2 tablespoons fresh lime juice (from 1 lime)

1. Preheat the oven to 400°F.

2. In a large bowl, place the cornmeal, almond flour, oat flour, ground flaxseed, baking powder, salt, and cumin (if using) and whisk together to blend.

3. Add the milk and lime juice, and knead lightly with your hands into a stringy but not sticky dough.

4. To make a large pizza: Spread a large sheet of parchment paper on a clean work surface. Sprinkle some cornmeal on it. Transfer the dough to the parchment and use a rolling pin to roll it out to a ¼-inch-thick 9 × 13-inch rectangle. Use your hands to lightly push the dough in around the perimeter and build up a slight edge. Slide the parchment paper with the crust onto the baking sheet. To make mini pizzas: Line two baking sheets with parchment paper. Divide the dough into 6 equal portions. Dust a clean work surface with cornmeal and roll out one portion into a 5-inch disk. Transfer to one of the prepared baking sheets, building up a slight edge to create a little height, if desired. Repeat with the remaining 5 portions.

5. Using a pastry brush or a spatula, lightly brush the top of the crust(s) with a little milk. Bake until the top of the crust(s) is dry and a little crisp, 15 to 20 minutes.

6. Remove from the oven and top with your desired pizza sauce and toppings, and bake again until the toppings are cooked, about 20 minutes.

RECIPES

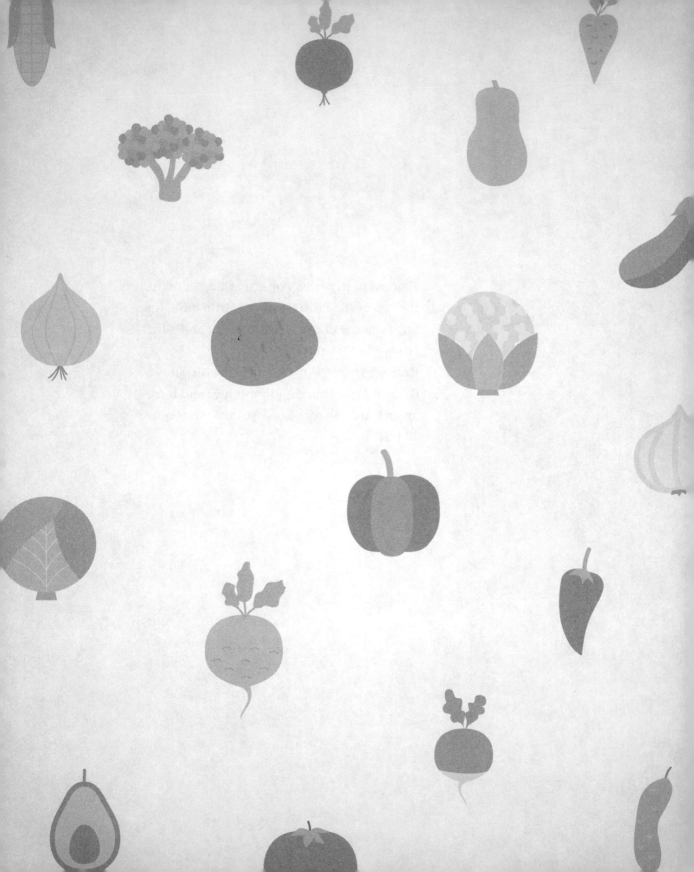

Acknowledgments

Thank you to the following individuals without whose contributions and support this book would not have been written: Brian Wendel and the rest of the Forks Over Knives team, thank you for continuing to give us such amazing opportunities, for your ongoing support, and for your cherished friendship. We admire your mission to make the world a healthier place and are honored for every occasion we get to partner with you. Thank you to Marah Stets for your collaboration and help in bringing this book to fruition. Thank you to Darshana Thacker; you make eating this way seductive—easy, extremely delicious, *and* health promoting! Thank you to Michelle Howry and the Touchstone team for championing our efforts and giving us a forum for sharing our thoughts with so many others.

And, finally, thank you to our families—you continue to inspire us daily to do what we do. We so appreciate your belief in us, support of us, and love for us! We love you all and wouldn't be here without you!

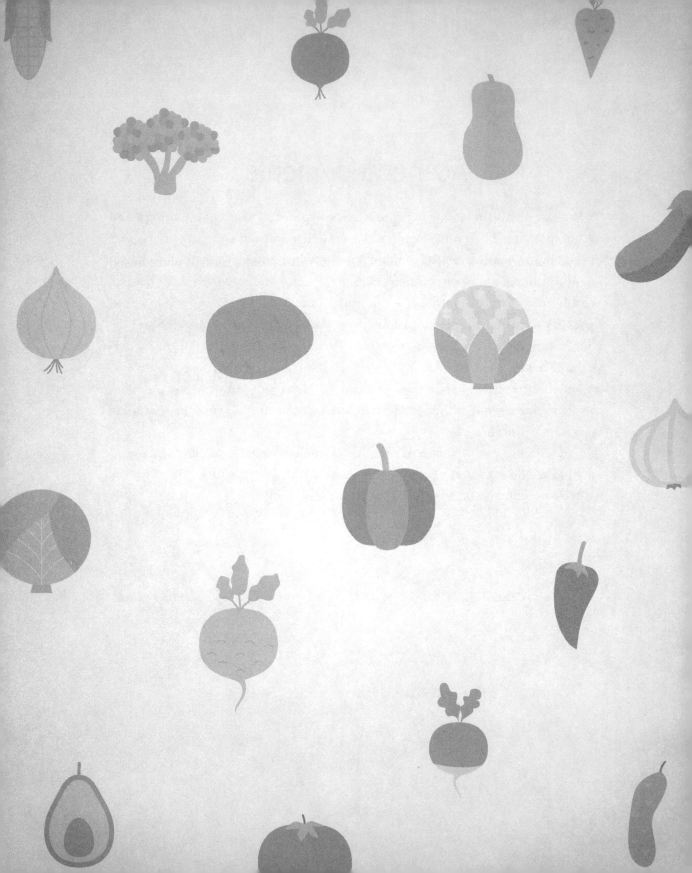

Resources

TO LEARN MORE

For more information or to become actively involved in the field of plant-based nutrition, check out these websites:

- 2Forks events: www.2forksevents.com

- Dr. McDougall's Health and Medical Center: www.drmcdougall.com

- Engine 2 Diet: www.engine2diet.com

- Forks Over Knives: www.forksoverknives.com

- Happy Cow, the Healthy Eating Guide: www.happycow.net

- Jeff Novick, MS, RD: www.JeffNovick.com

- Physicians Committee for Responsible Medicine: www.pcrm.org

- Dr. Esselstyn's Prevent and Reverse Heart Disease Program: www.heartattackproof.com

- T. Colin Campbell Center for Nutrition Studies: www.nutritionstudies.org

- TrueNorth Health Center: www.healthpromoting.com

- Wellness Forum Health: www.wellnessforum.com

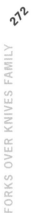

BOOKSHELF

Following are some essential books for the plant-based bibliophile:

- *21-Day Weight-Loss Kickstart* by Neal D. Barnard, MD, Grand Central, 2011.

- *Bravo!: Health-Promoting Meals from the TrueNorth Kitchen* by Ramses Bravo, Book Publishing Company, 2012.

- *Breaking the Food Seduction* by Neal D. Barnard, MD, St. Martin's Press, 2003.

- *Chef Del's Better Than Vegan* by Del Sroufe with Glen Merzer, BenBella Books, 2013.

- *China Study Cookbook* by LeAnne Campbell, PhD, BenBella Books, 2013.

- *Dr. McDougall's Digestive Tune-Up* by John A. McDougall, MD, Healthy Living Publications, 2006.

- *Dr. Neal Barnard's Program for Reversing Diabetes* by Neal D. Barnard, MD, Rodale, 2007.

- *Forks Over Knives—The Cookbook* by Del Sroufe, The Experiment, 2011.

- *Forks Over Knives: The Plant-Based Way to Health* by Gene Stone (ed.), The Experiment, 2011.

- *How Not to Die* by Michael Greger, MD, with Gene Stone, Flatiron Books, 2015.

- *Keep It Simple, Keep It Whole* by Alona Pulde, MD, and Matthew Lederman, MD, Exsalus Health & Wellness Center, 2009.

- *Plant-Strong* by Rip Esselstyn, Grand Central Life & Style, 2015.

- *Power Foods for the Brain* by Neal Barnard, Grand Central Life & Style, 2013.

- *Prevent and Reverse Heart Disease* by Caldwell B. Esselstyn Jr., MD, Avery Books, 2007.

- *The Campbell Plan* by Thomas Campbell, MD, Rodale Press, 2015.

- *The China Study* by T. Colin Campbell, PhD, and Thomas M. Campbell II, BenBella Books, 2006.

- *The Engine 2 Diet* by Rip Esselstyn, Grand Central Books, 2009.

- *The Forks Over Knives Plan* by Alona Pulde, MD, and Matthew Lederman, MD, Touchstone, 2014.

- *The McDougall Program for Maximum Weight Loss* by John McDougall, MD, Plume, 1995.

- *The McDougall Program: 12 Days to Dynamic Health* by John A. McDougall, MD, Plume, 1991.

- *The McDougall Quick & Easy Cookbook* by John A. McDougall, MD, and Mary McDougall, Plume, 1999.

- *The New McDougall Cookbook* by John McDougall, MD, and Mary McDougall, Plume, 1997.

- *Plant-Powered Families* by Dreena Burton, BenBella Books, 2015.

- *The Pleasure Trap* by Douglas J. Lisle, PhD, and Alan Goldhamer, DC, Book Publishing Company, 2006.

- *The Prevent and Reverse Heart Disease Cookbook* by Ann Crile Esselstyn and Jane Esselstyn, Avery, 2014.

- *The Starch Solution* by John A. McDougall, MD, and Mary McDougall, Rodale Books, 2012.

- *Whole: Rethinking the Science of Nutrition* by T. Colin Campbell, PhD, with Howard Jacobson, PhD, BenBella Books, 2013.

KIDS' BOOKSHELF

- Mitch Spinach book series by Hillary Feerick and Jeff Hillenbrand, illustrated by Andrea Vitali, Mitch Spinach Productions (www.mitchspinach.com).

- *Harmony on the Farm* by Sean R. Smith, illustrated by Jess Yeomans, CreateSpace Publishing, 2012.

DVDS

- *Forks Over Knives*, Virgil Films and Entertainment, 2011.

- *Forks Over Knives—The Extended Interviews*, Virgil Films and Entertainment, 2013.

- *Losing Weight Without Losing Your Mind* by Doug Lisle, PhD, John & Mary McDougall Productions, 2007.

- *The Pleasure Trap* by Doug Lisle, PhD, John & Mary McDougall Productions, 2004.

- *The Willpower Paradox* by Doug Lisle, PhD, John & Mary McDougall Productions, 2013.

- An assortment of nutrition DVDs available at www.jeffnovick.com

COURSES

- eCornell Certificate in Plant-Based Nutrition: www.nutritionstudies.org

- The Forks Over Knives Online Cooking Course

- The Starch Solution Certification Course: www.drmcdougall.com

MEAL PLANNING

- The Forks Meal Planner: www.forksmealplanner.com

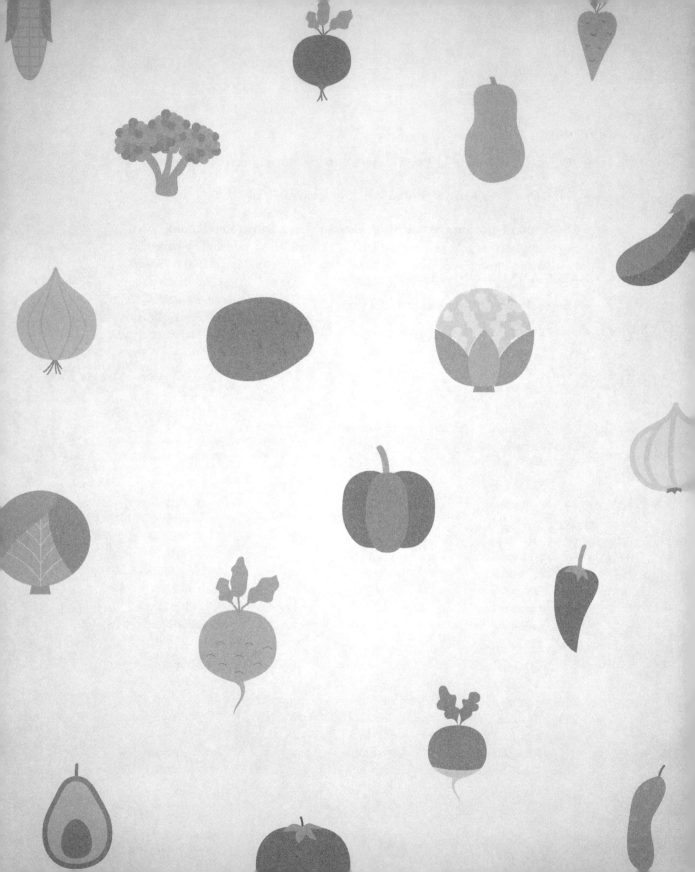

Notes

1. Maren Hegsted, Sally A. Schuette, Michael B. Zemel, and Hellen M. Linkswiler, "Urinary Calcium and Calcium Balance in Young Men as Affected by Level of Protein and Phosphorus Intake," *Journal of Nutrition* 111 (March 1981): 553–62; D. Joe Millward, "The Nutritional Value of Plant-Based Diets in Relation to Human Amino Acid and Protein Requirements," *Proceedings of the Nutritional Society* 58 (May 1999): 249–60; Eric C. Westman, William S. Yancy, Joel S. Edman, Keith F. Tomlin, and Christine E. Perkins, "Effect of 6-Month Adherence to a Very Low Carbohydrate Diet Program," *American Journal of Medicine* 113 (July 2002): 30–36; R. Itoh and Y. Suyama, "Sodium Excretion in Relation to Calcium and Hydroxyproline Excretion in a Healthy Japanese Population," *American Journal of Clinical Nutrition* 63 (May 1996): 735–40.

2. Amy Joy Lanou, "Should Dairy Be Recommended as Part of a Healthy Vegetarian Diet? Counterpoint," *American Journal of Clinical Nutrition* 89 (May 2009): 1638S–42S.

3. Allen S. Levine, Catherine M. Kotz, and Blake A. Gosnell, "Sugars: Hedonic Aspects, Neuroregulation, and Energy Balance," *American Journal of Clinical Nutrition* 78 (October 2003): 834S–42S; Barbara A. Smith, Thomas J. Fillion, and Elliott M. Blass, "Orally Mediated Sources of Calming in 1- to 3-Day-Old Human Infants," *Developmental Psychology* [serial online] 26 (September 1, 1990): 731–37; Elliot M. Blass and Vivian Ciaramitaro, "A New Look at Some Old Mechanisms in Human Newborns: Taste and Tactile Determinants of State, Affect, and Action," *Monographs of the Society of Research in Child Development* 59, no. 1 (1994): i–v, 1–81; Pamela J. Brink, "Addiction to Sugar," *Western Journal of Nursing Research* 15 (June 1993): 280–81.

4. Qi Sun, Donna Spiegelman, Rob M. van Dam, Michelle D. Holmes, Vasanti S. Malik, Walter C. Willett, Frank B. Hu, "White Rice, Brown Rice, and Risk of Type 2 Diabetes in U.S. Men and Women," *Archives of Internal Medicine* 170 (June 14, 2010): 961–69; Guillermo Llanos and Ingrid Libman, "Diabetes in the Americas," *Bulletin of the Pan American Health Organization* 28 (December 1994): 285–301; Teruo Kitagawa, Misao Owada, Tatsuhiko Urakami, and Kuniaki Yamauchi, "Increased Incidence of Non-Insulin Dependent Diabetes Mellitus Among

Japanese Schoolchildren Correlates with an Increased Intake of Animal Protein and Fat," *Clinical Pediatrics* 37 (February 1998): 111–15; Sok-Ja Janket, JoAnn E. Manson, Howard Sesso, Julie E. Buring, and Simin Liu, "A Prospective Study of Sugar Intake and Risk of Type 2 Diabetes in Women," *Diabetes Care* 26 (April 2003): 1008–15; Lawrence de Koning, Teresa T. Fung, Xiaomei Liao, et al., "Low-Carbohydrate Diet Scores and Risk of Type 2 Diabetes in Men," *American Journal of Clinical Nutrition* 93 (April 2011): 844–50.

5. K. J. I. Carpenter, "A Short History of Nutritional Science: Part 2 (1885–1912)," *Journal of Nutrition* 133, no. 4 (April 2003): 975–84.

6. M. Ebbing et al., "Cancer Incidence and Mortality After Treatment with Folic Acid and Vitamin B_{12}," *Journal of the American Medical Association* 302, no. 19 (November 18, 2009): 2119–26.

7. G. I. Bjelakovic, D. Nikolova, L. L. Gluud, R. G. Simonetti, and C. Gluud, "Mortality in Randomized Trials of Antioxidant Supplements for Primary and Secondary Prevention: Systematic Review and Meta-analysis," *Journal of the American Medical Association* 297, no. 8 (February 28, 2007): 842–57.

8. M. Suvi, Esa Läärä Vertanen, Elina Hyppönen, et al., "Cow's Milk Consumption, HLA-DQB1 Genotype, and Type 1 Diabetes: A Nested Case-Control Study of Siblings of Children with Diabetes," *Diabetes* 49 (June 2000): 912–17; American Academy of Pediatrics Work Group on Cow's Milk Protein and Diabetes Mellitus, "Infant Feeding Practices and Their Possible Relationship to the Etiology of Diabetes Mellitus," *Pediatrics* 94 (November 1, 1994): 752–54; Jukka Karjalainen, Julio M. Martin, Mikael Knip, et al., "A Bovine Albumin Peptide as a Possible Trigger of Insulin-Dependent Diabetes Mellitus," *New England Journal of Medicine* 327 (July 30, 1992): 302–7.

9. C. Adebamowo et al., "High School Dietary Dairy Intake and Teenage Acne," *Journal of the American Academy of Dermatology* 52, no. 2 (February 2005): 207–14; G. Iacono et al., "Intolerance of Cow's Milk and Chronic Constipation in Children," *New England Journal of Medicine* 339, no. 16 (October 1998): 1100–104.

10. Jim Bartley and Susan Read McGlashan, "Does Milk Increase Mucus Production?" *Medical Hypotheses* 74 (April 2010): 732–34; John A. Jenkins, Heimo Breiteneder, and E. N. Clare Mills, "Evolutionary Distance from Human Homologs Reflects Allergenicity of Animal Food Proteins," *Journal of Allergy and Clinical Immunology* 120 (December 2007): 1399–405; D. C. Heiner, "Respiratory Diseases and Food Allergy," *Annals of Allergy, Asthma & Immunology* 53, no. 6, part 2

(December 1984): 657–64; J. Cant, "Food Allergy in Childhood," *Human Nutrition–Applied Nutrition* 39 (August 1985): 277–93.

11. D. M. Hegsted, "Calcium and Osteoporosis," *Journal of Nutrition* 116 (July 15, 1986): 2316–19.

12. Robert A. Vogel, Mary C. Corretti, and Gary D. Plotnick, "The Postprandial Effect of Components of the Mediterranean Diet on Endothelial Function," *Journal of the American College of Cardiology* 36 (November 1, 2000): 1455–60; David H. Blankenhorn, Ruth L. Johnson, Wendy J. Mack, Hafez A. El Zein, and Laura I. Vailas, "The Influence of Diet on the Appearance of New Lesions in Human Coronary Arteries," *Journal of the American Medical Association* 263 (March 23, 1990): 1646–52.

13. D. C. E. Nordström, C. Friman, Y. T. Konttinen, V. E. A. Honkanen, Y. Nasu, and E. Antila, "Alpha-Linolenic Acid in the Treatment of Rheumatoid Arthritis. A Double-Blind, Placebo-Controlled and Randomized Study: Flaxseed vs. Safflower Seed," *Rheumatology International* 14 (1995): 231–34; M. A. Allman, M. M. Pena, and D. Pang, "Supplementation with Flaxseed Oil Versus Sunflowerseed Oil in Healthy Young Men Consuming a Low-Fat Diet: Effects on Platelet Composition and Function," *European Journal of Clinical Nutrition* 49 (March 1995): 169–78; M. R. Namazi, "The Beneficial and Detrimental Effects of Linoleic Acid on Autoimmune Disorders," *Autoimmunity* 37 (February 2004): 73–75; P. Purasiri, A. McKechnie, S. D. Heys, and O. Eremin, "Modulation in Vitro of Human Natural Cytotoxicity, Lymphocyte Proliferative Response to Mitogens and Cytokine Production by Essential Fatty Acids," *Immunology* 92 (October 1997): 166–72; D. Hazlett, "Dietary Fats Appear to Reduce Lung Function," *Journal of the American Medical Association* 223, no. 1 (1973): 15–16; Clifford W. Welsch, "Relationship Between Dietary Fat and Experimental Mammary Tumorigenesis: A Review and Critique," *Cancer Research* 52 (April 1992): 2040S–48S; Patrizia Griffini, Olav Fehres, Lars Klieverik, et al., "Dietary Omega-3 Polyunsaturated Fatty Acids Promote Colon Carcinoma Metastasis in Rat Liver," *Cancer Research* 58 (August 1, 1998): 3312–19; Lars Klieverik, Olav Fehres, Patrizia Griffini, Cornelis J. F. Van Noorden, and Wilma M. Frederiks, "Promotion of Colon Cancer Metastases in Rat Liver by Fish Oil Diet Is Not Due to Reduced Stroma Formation," *Clinical & Experimental Metastasis* 18 (September 2000): 371–77; Kenneth K. Karroll, "Experimental Evidence of Dietary Factors and Hormone-Dependent Cancers," *Cancer Research* 35 (November 1975): 3374–83; J. H. Weisburger, "Worldwide Prevention of Cancer and Other Chronic Diseases Based on Knowledge of Mechanisms," *Mutation Research* 402 (June 18, 1998):

331–37; Leonard A. Sauer, David E. Blask, and Robert T. Bauchey, "Dietary Factors and Growth and Metabolism in Experimental Tumors," *Journal of Nutritional Biochemistry* 18 (October 2007): 637–49; Clement Ip, "Review of the Effects of Trans Fatty Acids, Oleic Acid, N-3 Polyunsaturated Fatty Acids, and Conjugated Linoleic Acid on Mammary Carcinogenesis in Animals," *American Journal of Clinical Nutrition* 66 (December 1997): 1523S–29S.

14. Susan A. New and D. Joe Millward, "Calcium, Protein, and Fruit and Vegetables as Dietary Determinants of Bone Health," *American Journal of Clinical Nutrition* 77 (May 2003): 1340–41; Thomas Remer and Friedrich Manz, "Potential Renal Acid Load of Foods and Its Influence on Urine pH," *Journal of the American Dietetic Association* 95 (July 1995): 791–97; Eva Warensjö, Liisa Byberg, Håkan Melhus, et al., "Dietary Calcium Intake and Risk of Fracture and Osteoporosis: Prospective Longitudinal Cohort Study," *BMJ* 342 (May 24, 2011): d1473; Morgan E. Levine, Jorge A. Suarez, Sebastian Brandhorst, et al., "Low Protein Intake Is Associated with a Major Reduction in IGF-1, Cancer, and Overall Mortality in the 65 and Younger but Not Older Population," *Cell Metabolism* 19 (March 4, 2014): 407–17.

Index

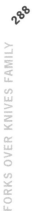